ALZHEIMER'S - DEMENTIA

Find the Best Nursing Home with Sister Ann

Ann Marie Gallogly

authorHOUSE

AuthorHouse™ UK
1663 Liberty Drive
Bloomington, IN 47403 USA
www.authorhouse.co.uk
Phone: 0800.197.4150

© 2015 Ann Marie Gallogly. All rights reserved.

No part of this book may be reproduced, stored in a retrieval system, or transmitted by any means without the written permission of the author.

Published by AuthorHouse 12/08/2015

ISBN: 978-1-5049-9585-6 (sc)
ISBN: 978-1-5049-9586-3 (hc)
ISBN: 978-1-5049-9587-0 (e)

Library of Congress Control Number: 2015920127

Print information available on the last page.

Any people depicted in stock imagery provided by Thinkstock are models, and such images are being used for illustrative purposes only. Certain stock imagery © Thinkstock.

This book is printed on acid-free paper.

Because of the dynamic nature of the Internet, any web addresses or links contained in this book may have changed since publication and may no longer be valid. The views expressed in this work are solely those of the author and do not necessarily reflect the views of the publisher, and the publisher hereby disclaims any responsibility for them.

Contents

Acknowledgement vii
Life History xi

Part 1

Nurse Ann's Profile 1
Introduction 5
Care Home Staff 9
Pre-Visit Information Guide 15
Pre-Visit: What to Look Out For 20
Your First Visit to the Home 48
Benefits of the Care/Nursing Home 85
My Mother 89
Nursing in Pre-Private-Nursing-Home Times 93
Testimonials 95

Part 2

A History of Dementia 101
Person-Centred Care (PCC) University Module 111

Epilogue	129
Author References	131
About the Author	139
About the Book	141

Acknowledgement

To my husband, Eamon, and our family (for keeping the fire lit) when I was working day or night duty. To all the staff and families of residents who supported me in gaining my nursing experience.

I loved my job and I loved you all.

To Chris, my first contact at AuthorHouse and all there who encouraged me to finish my book and so made this happen, and also to Willie for taking the images for me.

To everyone who suffers from Alzheimer's disease, and to their families.

Life History

I was born and reared in County Armagh, Northern Ireland. From an early age, I always had a desire to help people. My dream came true when I obtained my nursing qualifications and I began working.

I am happily married for over forty years, and we have four grown children who all still live close to us. My three grandchildren visit me every day.

All work and no play will make anyone a dull person, and I certainly did enjoy life outside work. When my family was young, my husband, our friends, and I took our families out every Sunday, and we cycled around the local area and visited places of historical interest. We cycled around Ireland and raised fourteen thousand pounds in aid of Ethiopia at the time of Live Aid. This activity continued until the kids grew up and went to university or followed their futures.

I still love to keep up with my close network of friends by going out for meals, dancing, attending concerts, holidays, and much more.

I do volunteer work for our local hospice since my sister died a few years ago. This gives me an opportunity to give something back to the hospice for the help they gave me and my family.

I am a keen reader, especially books by Michael Connolly and James Patterson. I learned to make Carrickmacross lace as a child and later in life held classes in my local area, teaching the craft.

I also enjoy making and giving Carrickmacross lace bridal and newborn presents for my family and friends. An example of these gifts is shown in the photograph below.

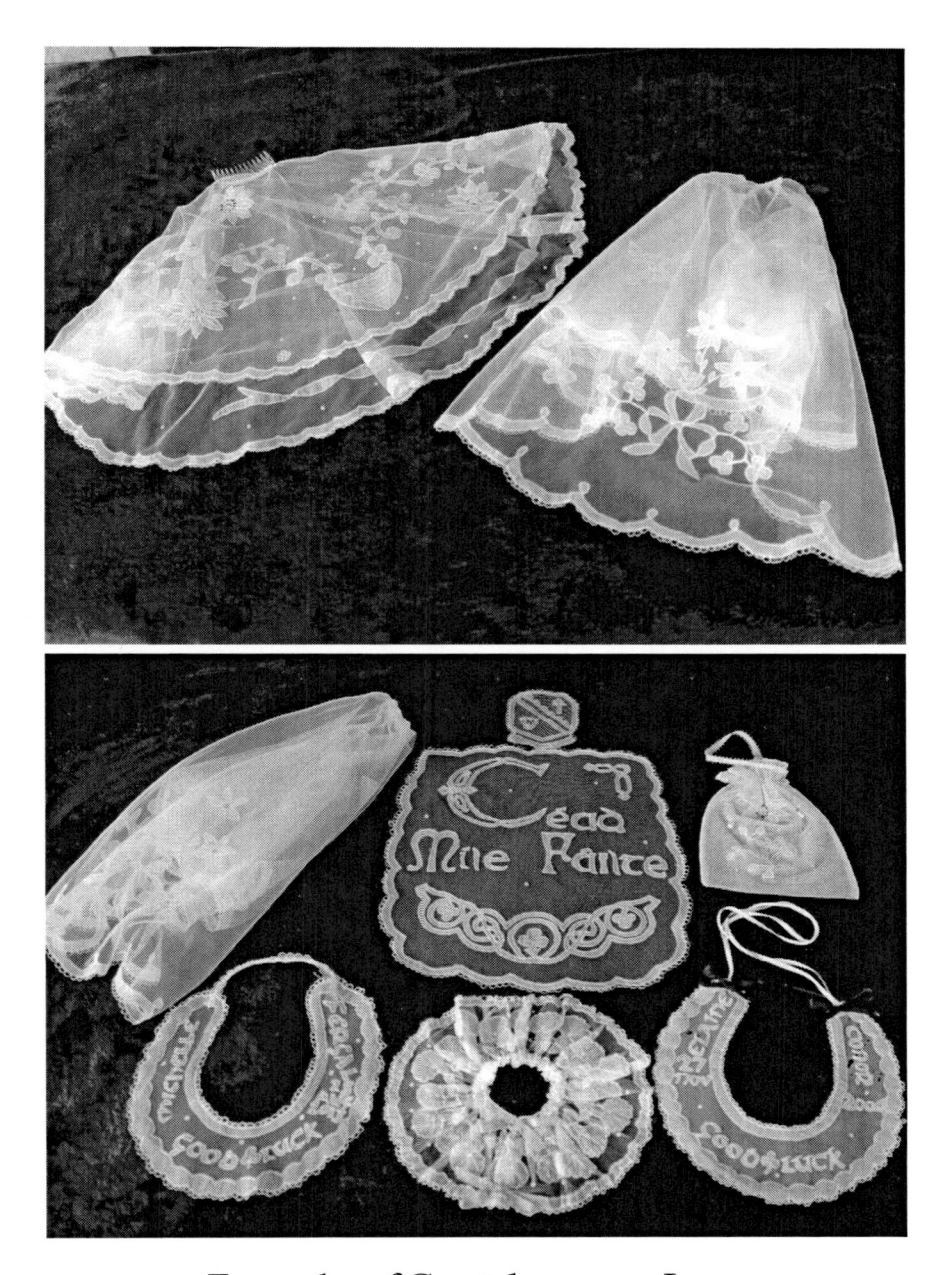

Examples of Carrickmacross Lace.

I now want to pass on my experiences and knowledge gained from my life working as a nurse to sufferers and families dealing with Alzheimer's disease, so I decided to write this book. I hope it will help those worried about Alzheimer's disease and give them an insight into what to expect if they or a family member should need to be admitted into a home. I hope it also benefits my own family, as well as student nurses, care assistants (especially overseas staff), or anyone working in an Alzheimer's home.

Part 1

Nurse Ann's Profile

I have been a practicing registered nurse for more than thirty years and have recently retired.

My main area of practice has been nursing residents in various care and nursing homes within the general area where I live. Positions I have held include Staff Nurse, Sister, and Manager. I have extensive experience in caring for those suffering from Alzheimer's disease.

My professional experience has given me great insight into the different cultures and backgrounds of both Residents and Staff. My colleagues have included nurses and nursing assistants/carers from several continents, who have enriched my understanding of people across the world, and they in turn enriched my life and the residents' lives also.

My experience has given me invaluable insight into different cultures and has taught me what overseas staff need to know in order to care for dementia patients here. I have also learnt from them how to care for someone from overseas too.

Nursing qualifications and experience include:

- training to become a registered general nurse
- training in employing all staff
- training in vulnerable adults, abuse, health and safety, moving and handling, challenging behaviour, and pain, to name just a few
- training for trainers – Alzheimer's course whereby she has been trained to train all staff in the understanding and caring for Alzheimer's residents
- training in communication in dementia
- university module in dementia/Alzheimer's

My training, along with my practical nursing, has equipped me to teach by example how to care for vulnerable people.

Like Florence Nightingale, I feel nursing hands-on is still the best means of knowing people's needs and taking care of them.

I believe it is the same the world over. We nurses care for our patients and know when to be their advocate when they need us, especially when they are elderly, sick, and vulnerable.

I make sure to know the residents' personalities, likes, and dislikes, as do the other members of the staff. This is what nursing is all about.

Introduction

If you need help and advice on choosing a care home for your loved one, I hope this book will help you.

Do you know what goes on behind the closed front door of a care home? Do you know how to recognise good care in a care home, especially an Alzheimer's care home? Do you know what is good versus bad practice in feeding, personal care, environment, dealing with challenging behaviour, pain relief, and sedation? Would you recognise abuse in the care home? If your answer to any of these questions is no, then this book will be of invaluable help to you.

I have worked as a trained nurse in the caring profession for thirty years, and I want to pass on to you the inside knowledge and experience I have gained. Firstly, I want to inform my own nearest and dearest how I would want to be cared for if the time comes for me to be admitted into a care home. and secondly, *you* need to know too.

I will share with you my knowledge and advice, to help you make an informed decision on the choices ahead. This will be based on my years working inside the profession on a daily basis and understanding the fears you have about your loved one's future. You may have read horror stories about homes in the news, so I felt it was time to inform the public of what I believe is right and wrong in providing care to the vulnerable and what to look out for when first visiting care homes.

When entering the nursing home, you must use all your senses to evaluate the standard of home you are visiting. Go beyond simply looking; pay attention to sounds and smells as well.

You will discover why the environment, communication, and activities are crucial to the physical and mental well-being of the person suffering from dementia of any sort.

I will discuss important issues, pain, challenging behaviour (also called distress reaction), abuse, restraint, and weight loss; its causes; and how it should be dealt with.

After reading this information, with all the situations that can arise in a nursing home, it should help you make an informed decision on what is a good home and what is not.

I know the qualifications necessary for each staff member. I have always expected dignity, respect, and privacy to be showered on the residents at all times and have trained the staff according to my high standards.

In closing, I will point out that I believe most homes are well run and regulated by the authorities, but when there is no inspection on or no visitors to see, that's when you need to trust the home and **not worry about the closed front door.**

Care Home Staff

Trained Nursing Staff:

Professionally trained staff include nurse manager/deputy, administrator, sister, staff nurses.

Ancillary Staff:

Ancillary staff include nursing carers, activities coordinator, administrator, cook and cooking assistants, domestic, cleaning and laundry staff, and the maintenance person who ensures the safety of the building on a daily basis.

Outside Professionals:

These professionals contribute to the overall care of the residents: tissue viability specialist, occupational therapist, speech and language therapist, own doctor (GP) and consultant dietician, dental and optical specialists, to name but a few.

Staff (Brief) Job Descriptions:

The home manager/deputy:

He or she sets the standard of care for the home. The manager knows the type of personality of a person suitable to work with people suffering from Alzheimer's disease. They take this into account at the interview stage, and whether the interviewee has experience or not is irrelevant. (They can be trained in the home to their standards.)

Each manager makes the decision whether to employ someone based on a police check, together with previous references and the results of the interview.

Everyone in the home should have training in working with people with Alzheimer's disease, whether it be the cook, domestic, laundry, maintenance staff, or activities coordinator, and especially all nursing and caring staff. This makes it easier for the person with Alzheimer's to be understood, and communication is enhanced.

The Sister/Charge Nurse:

He or she ensures proper care is carried out by overseeing the training and support of nursing staff. He or she has a more personal relationship with the resident and family and is most likely the family's first point of contact; he or she endeavours to carry out the family's wishes.

The charge nurse ensures the smooth day-to-day organisation of the unit by overseeing all nursing and non-nursing duties, namely cleaning, laundry, maintenance of the building and equipment, to name but a few, liaising with families and outside professionals whilst being answerable to the manager.

The Nurse:

He or she carries out detailed care plans for each resident, and a primary nurse is identified for each resident, to oversee the care she has planned. Each resident is allocated a separate nurse who makes out the individual care plan and instructs each staff member through the care plan, showing how this resident should be cared for. In essence, the sister and nurse's duties are being responsible for the day-to-day personal care provided to the resident.

Care Assistants:

When someone requires total nursing care, his or her basic care requirements are the same, no matter what disease he or she suffers from.

What is required is that the staff have specialised training in dementia care. This is to ensure that all staff understand the mental requirements of the person suffering from Alzheimer's, along with the resident's physical requirements.

The carer/nursing assistant's role is to provide care for the very basic everyday physical functions of the body, e.g., toileting, washing, dressing, eating, and drinking. The carer is one of the most important people in the resident's life now – except for you, the family, of course. The carer and the person with Alzheimer's form an attachment with each other. Therefore, the carer is more likely to be the first person to know when something is wrong with the resident. Any problems that are found are then reported to the nurse.

Fully trained nursing care assistants are essential to the physical and mental health of the resident. The senior carer/nursing assistant is the person who takes instructions from the sister/nurse and ensures the other carers on the floor carry out the instructions required. As you can see, there is a process whereby the resident's needs are communicated from each group of staff; it is teamwork throughout.

Ann Marie Gallogly

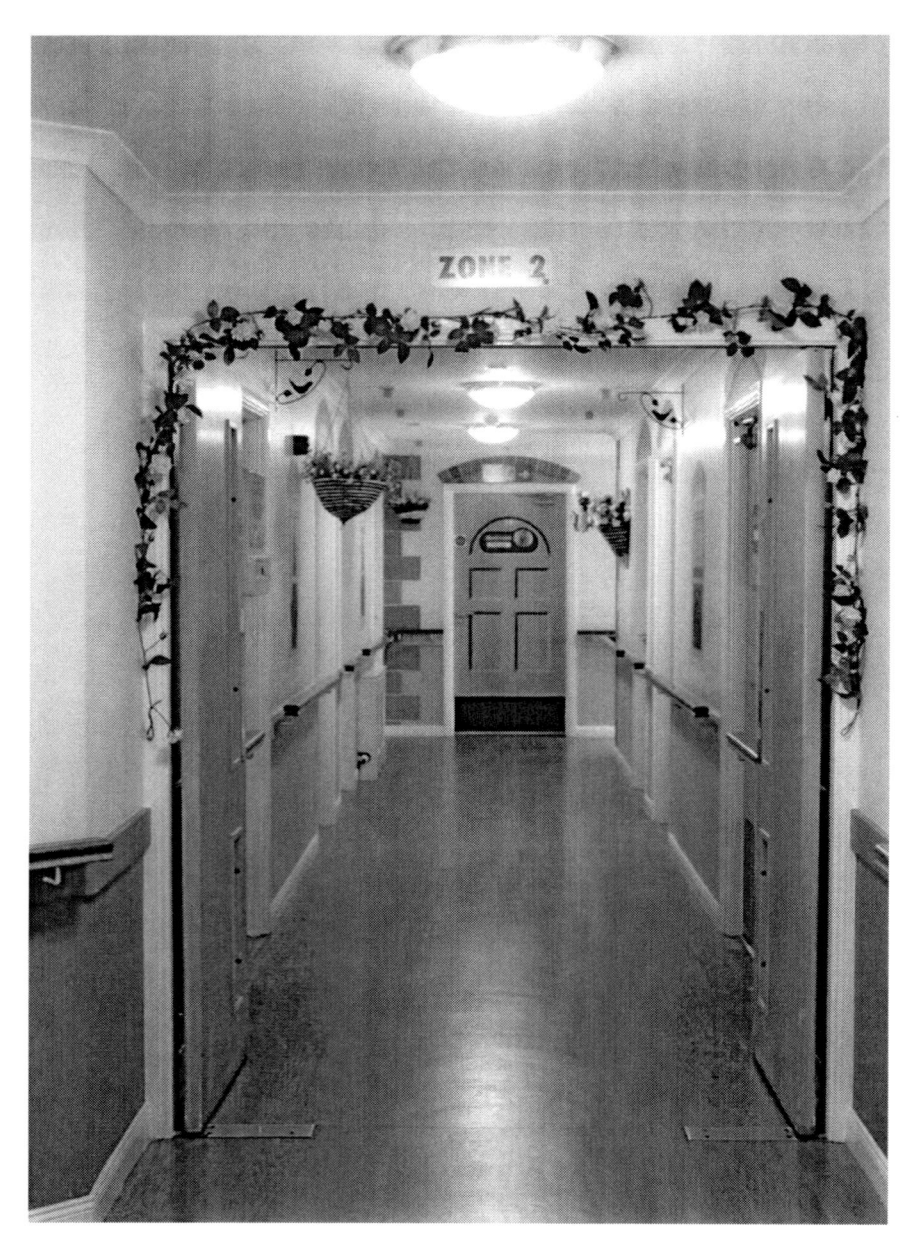

Welcome to the Home.

Pre-Visit Information Guide

This part of the book is a nursing sister's inside-information guide on what to look out for when choosing a nursing home for your loved one who is experiencing Alzheimer's disease (or any type of dementia). This information is important to know before visiting any potential care homes.

We have all read in newspapers about good homes versus bad homes, but really it is the people running the home or the people working in the home that the question is about. If it a government-run home or a privately run home, it should make no difference. There are statistics for each type of home, and in each country the figures differ.

To me, it is the people who are working in the home who have the influence to change a potential bad situation to a good one. Nurses have a duty of care to the people they nurse, and they have the power to influence their employers in the services they supply.

Thankfully the good homes outnumber the bad homes, but even one bad home is one too many. You will see from the following inside information what should be expected in a good home and what should be provided to the resident.

Please do not feel guilty for having to place your loved one in a nursing home. It is the most difficult decision you are about to make, but it is made in the best interests of your loved one and yourself. I have seen families tearing themselves apart over the guilt. You have done all you can; now you need further help.

For ease of reading, I'm going to name this next resident Joe.

At this point, Joe has had all the tests and has been diagnosed with Alzheimer's disease. You have lived with the deterioration in his physical and mental condition and cannot cope any longer. You may feel the change has made him unrecognisable.

He may have had a personality change from being a quiet, reserved personality to someone who shouts abuse, and maybe he becomes physically aggressive when he is distressed. Joe may walk about all the time or get cross and become physical when he cannot perform a simple task. Maybe the police had to bring him home from town one day, as he did not recognise where he was, or because of his short-term memory, he has forgotten who you are, calling you his brother and not recognising you as his son.

Perhaps he becomes disoriented and confused or he is at risk in the house, leaving the cooker on or forgetting how or when to turn it off. Maybe he is always afraid of being on his own and needs your company all the time, or he is always looking home, but you know the home he is looking for is in the past, with his parents. It's just not possible to recreate the past.

Maybe it's a combination of all these factors. He is afraid of what is happening to him; he knows something is wrong but can't understand it. Fear is a big part of his life now. He now needs twenty-four-hour care and help from professionals.

You are exhausted by the constant worry of looking after him, so you need this help. Fear is a big part of your life too.

Be reassured – there is help for you too. Staff in these homes for people who are suffering from Alzheimer's should be trained in handling all situations, but you as a family can also play an important part in your loved one's care. I will guide you in what to look for in choosing a suitable home for Joe.

The location may be the key element so you and his friends can visit. Ultimately it may be only family visiting, as friends sometimes cannot handle the change in Joe. (This is what I have observed through the years.)

You will be armed with information from Joe's social worker and can research great Alzheimer's sites on the Internet, but I feel they do not cover all the types of questions I would ask and the answers to expect if I were considering admitting my loved one into a care home environment.

To me, it is the small things that count. Read closely what I have to suggest.

Visit as many homes in the area as possible – the best care and safety facilities, provided by the best-trained staff within a reasonable distance from your home.

When admitting Joe to a home, your first choice may not be available, so he may have to be admitted to your second choice and go on the waiting list for a bed in the first-choice home. You will need to inform the manager that Joe may only be there short term until the bed in your first-choice home becomes available. However, you never know – the second-choice home may turn out to be the best after all. Then you will not have to decide again.

I will not discuss the financial aspects, only the nursing issues, as this is my area of expertise.

Pre-Visit: What to Look Out For

Before going to visit the home for the first time, do a little research, so you will recognise for yourself the services the home can and should provide. In this chapter, we will look into location, décor of unit, trained staff, nursing care, pain, activities, and abuse, so you know what to look out for.

It should be obvious to the layman that with the décor and atmosphere of the home, the management is catering to the needs of the people experiencing Alzheimer's disease and staff suitably qualified to carry out the care.

Location:

The location depends on where you live, keeping in mind if you are planning to visit regularly or not. When you have done your homework on the type of home required and you have visited and examined the homes on your list, this will determine the location.

The nursing care home should be a setting like home away from home, only more secure, with code locks on the doors and gates to prevent anyone walking into the outside world, where they may get lost. Although inside the building, the residents should be free to walk about anywhere they wish, as long as it is safe to do so.

A person may settle in on the first day, but sometimes it can take several weeks. During this time, the resident and family members become familiar with the staff and the surroundings. The staff are trained to help the resident relax, and they communicate to each other in their own specific way. The family find it very hard to let go sometimes, and they also need reassuring as to the loved one's feelings. It is very hard for the family when the resident wants to go home with them after a visit. This is when the staff can help by distracting the resident with an activity that he or she likes.

It is difficult to admit, but it is sometimes a blessing that the short-term-memory loss enables the resident to forget that the family has gone home. However, the family goes home worried and concerned about their loved one and often rings the home in tears, enquiring about him or her. At this point, I am able to reassure them that Joe has forgotten the incident and he is now sitting, having his tea or whatever he is actually doing. Nurses understand the pressure on families and the guilt feelings they may have. I discuss this in more detail later in this book.

A great nursing home, wherever the location, will support the family and keep them informed at all times of any concerns they have about their loved one.

Alzheimer's - Dementia

Photograph of a Store.

Décor of Unit:

The actual planning of the colour scheme should be well planned, keeping the thoughts and feelings of Alzheimer's sufferers in mind.

The picture of the store above, with the name on the door, identifies it as a place of danger. Notice the top of the door and the upper wall are painted one colour, and the bottom half of the door and walls are painted a different colour. This is done on purpose, so as to make the door less obvious to the resident.

Exit doors are painted the same colour and style as the walls, to make the exit doors less obvious too. The residents would sometimes stand at the exit door, looking to get out (if the door was painted in a contrasting colour), and this can be very frustrating for them, thus leading to challenging behaviour and also making it very difficult to let anyone into the unit. The same thinking is used for doors leading to a laundry, electrical store, cleaning store, medicine room, or anywhere it would be dangerous for the resident to enter. Coded locks are also on these doors. Exit doors with panels should be of smoked glass, not clear glass, thus preventing anyone looking into the unit – and more importantly, anyone looking out. It is very sad if a resident watches a visitor leaving.

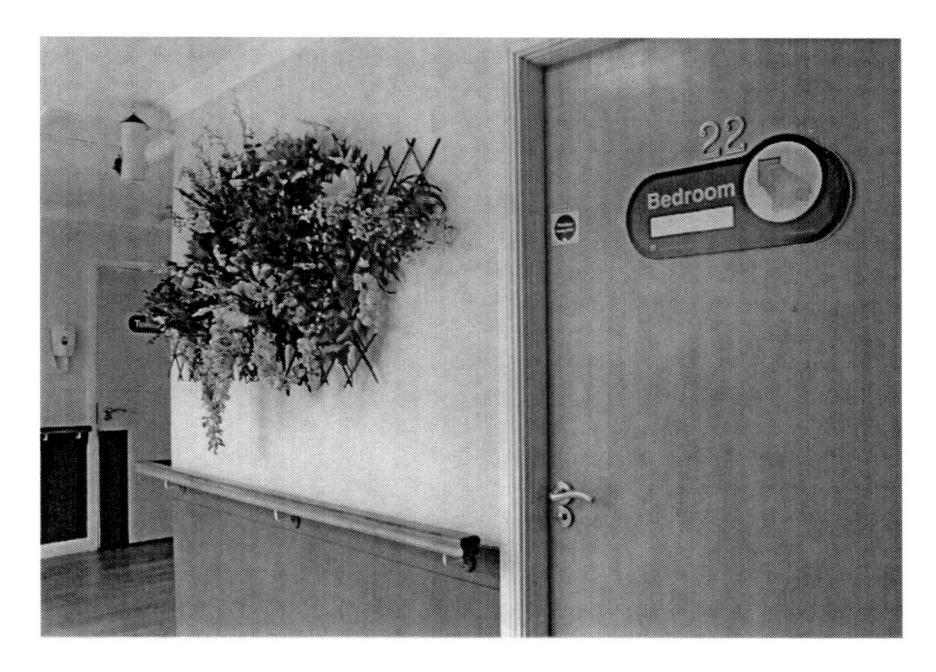

Photograph of a Bedroom.

The opposite is done for rooms the resident is free to enter. The bathroom, shower room, bedroom, and dining room are highlighted by using contrasting colours on the walls and doors. Notice the colour of the bedroom door above with the surrounding walls and handrail. A photo of the purpose of each room should be placed on the outside of the door – for example, a picture of a bath or shower; the name of a restaurant on the dining room; and of course the resident's name on his or her own bedroom door. A picture that they recognise of themselves, whether it be a present-day photo or one taken when they were younger, can also be inserted in a slot on the bedroom door; this can be decided between the resident and family.

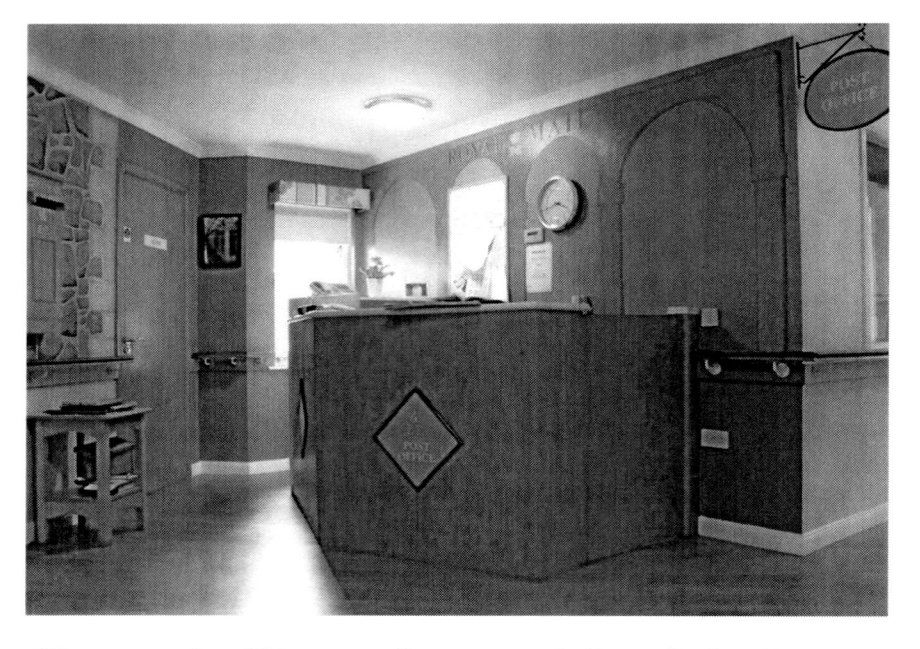

Photograph of Nursing Station with Post Office Design.

Decorating the nurses' station/office area as a post office, with all the signs attached to the post office, is a great reminder of the activity whereby the resident went to the post office every week to collect his or her retirement pension. This area is less clinical and more familiar and comforting to the resident.

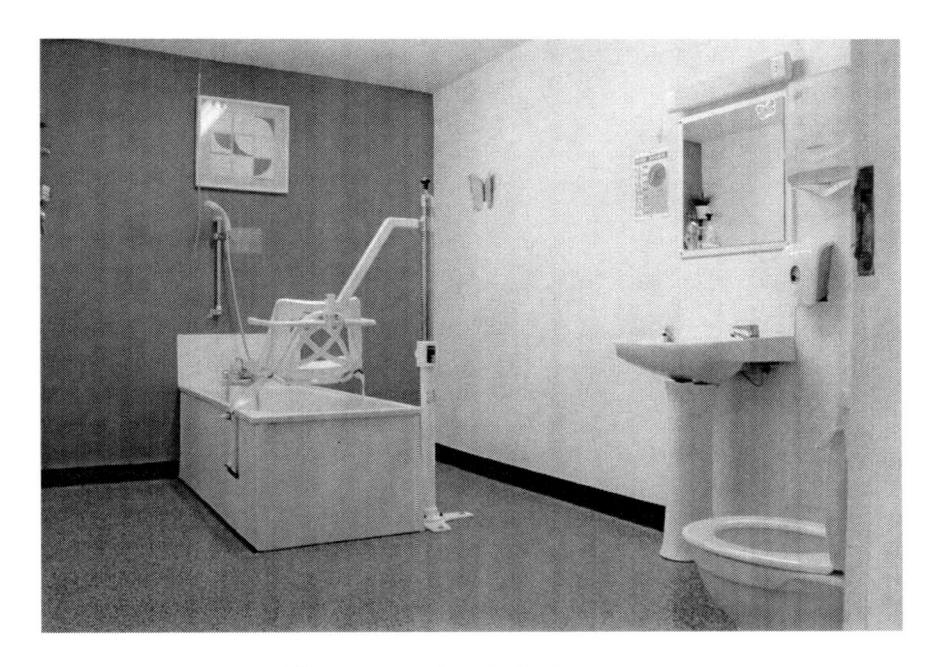

Photograph of Bathroom.

Ann Marie Gallogly

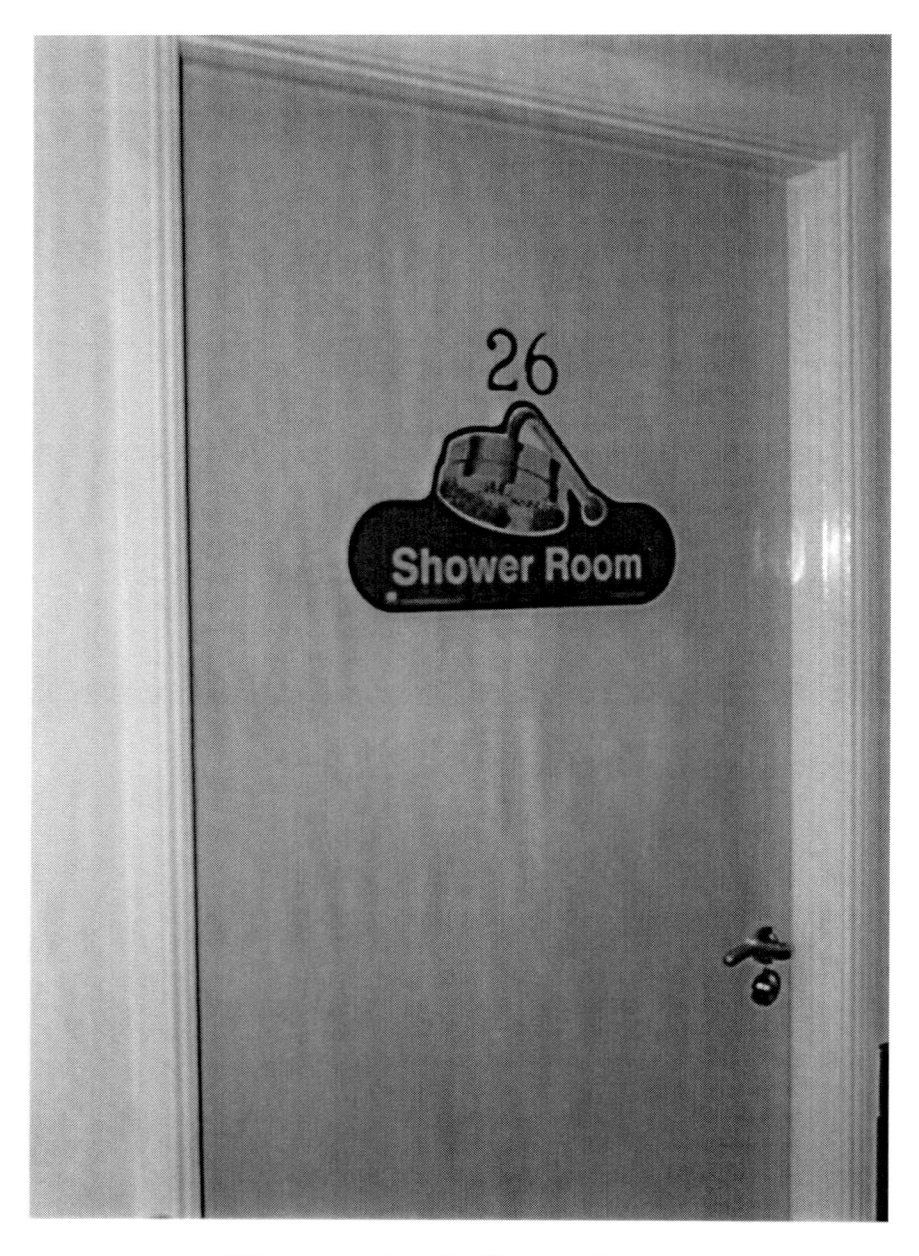

Photograph of a Shower Door.

Another area of thought and planning is the inside of the actual bathroom and shower room. Notice from the pictures above that the back wall is a different colour than the side walls, and the floor is a different colour still. This makes the toilet and bath more obvious, and the resident is reminded why he or she went in there in the first place. As per the above photograph of the shower door, the purpose of the room, in this case a shower room, is illustrated in writing, number, and in picture form on the outside too.

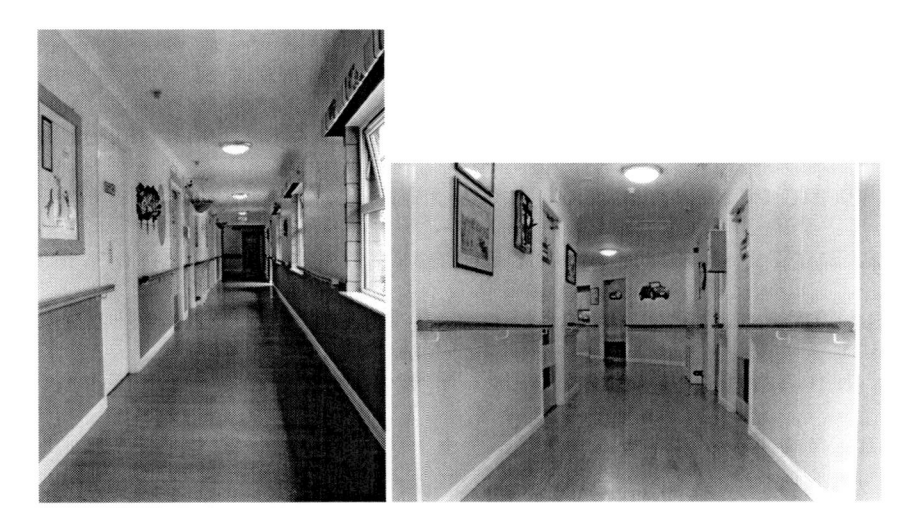

Photograph of Green Corridor.
Photograph of Orange Corridor.

The various corridors could be colour-coded. You can see from the two corridor pictures above that the lower wall on one corridor is yellow and the other corridor is green. This makes it easier for the residents to find their own room, as they may remember the colour of their corridor, rather than a specific room number.

Another design feature to help residents find the dining room is to rename it 'The Restaurant'. At home, the resident may have eaten on his or her own in the kitchen, and the transition to eating a meal in a large dining room with other people may feel alien to him or her. It would have felt normal in the past to share meals with others when dining in a restaurant. This may help the residents look forward to mealtimes in 'The Restaurant', especially if they are sitting in their favourite chair at the same table with the same resident beside them, as this creates a new feeling of familiarity at mealtimes for the residents. This is very important.

Alzheimer's - Dementia

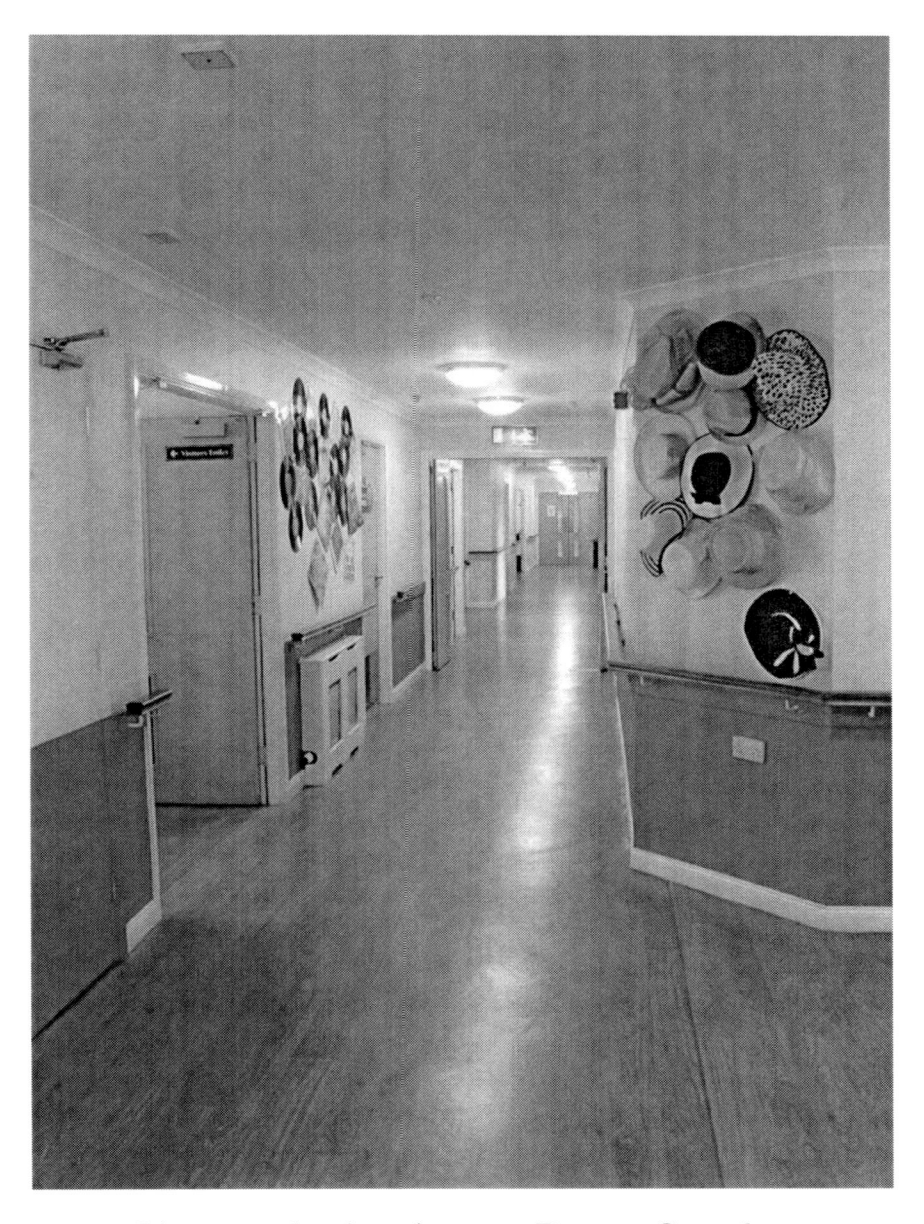

Photograph of an Activity Design Corridor.

Activities:

The above picture of an activity design corridor is designed to stimulate conversation between the residents themselves or the residents and families or staff. It creates an activity for the residents. They can look at the items, for example a hat, and then discuss if they like it, used to have one like it, or don't like it at all.

Any nursing/care home should have an activities person employed to stimulate the residents mentally and provide communication and relaxation when needed. This person should have specialised training in communication and have the necessary skill to recognise what activity would be suitable for each resident.

When walking about, observe closely what activities are arranged for the residents.

Activities play a major part in the resident's sense of feeling good and help when the resident is having a bad day. The activities need to be wide and varied to suit different interests and backgrounds. They need to be structured and written up on the notice board, so have a look at the notice board.

Check whether the planned activity is actually carried out at the time stated and that the board is updated regularly.

Observe whether the bedrooms are individual bedrooms and whether they reflect the residents individually. Do the rooms have personal possessions, photos of the resident's family, and pictures of the residents' personal interests in the room? These help the residents feel more at home and comfortable in their new surroundings and are a good sign.

Another good sign is if there is friendly interaction and chats between the staff and the residents.

Music and Exercise Therapy:
Singing, dancing, and using musical instruments is great fun, using family songs of their era. Some residents will have trouble remembering names and words when conversing, but put one of their favourite songs on, and they will sing along with the group.

Reminiscence and Recall/Life Story Work:
Reminiscence and recall therapy is based on the information gathered on admission from the resident's life story. Reminiscence therapy is a very interactive activity; it helps

residents to get to know one another, make friends, and recall memories.

In this therapy, props are used to help trigger residents' memories, allowing them to take part in the activity, which has good memories or feelings for them.

One of our activities people went to the local library and hired out books about old items of furniture, agricultural implements, irons, and many more articles. During the interactive activity session, the residents had a great discussion with each other and staff about the contents of the books. The conversation continued with the residents recognising the items, and everyone talked about how they were used. The residents knew more about the items than the activities person herself!

These props should include items that can stimulate the senses of smell, touch, sound, and sight.

Don't be afraid to ask the manager what aids the home supplies to assist this, for example memory boxes, old artefacts, and old photos of the local area.

Are there hairdressing, beauty, and relaxation services provided? Are they being carried out by trained therapists? Note that some relaxation techniques may not work for every resident.

Arts and Crafts:

Activities should be reflective of the residents' hobbies and interests, for example knitting, sewing, painting, and model-making. Doll therapy, as discussed later, works well for female residents when the need for comfort is evident.

Ask about the policy regarding bringing in pets for therapy, as not all homes allow pets into the building. The home may allow specially trained pet therapists to visit the home as an activity. Inform the manager if the resident has any allergies or fears of any animals.

How does the care home celebrate special occasions, for example, birthdays? You would need to know their procedure for this, as you may not be allowed to bring in your own birthday cake. The home may not be covered for insurance for outside catering.

Not all residents respond to or even like group therapy. Therefore, one-to-one activity may be required. An example is hand massage. This should be planned for and written up on the notice board.

Life Story Work:

This can be obtained at admission from the family, who will give the social history, likes and dislikes in relation to music, films, sport, dancing, and creative pastimes like gardening, knitting, sewing, or painting, to name a few.

Life story work should be carried out for each person and will help staff to get to know each resident, thus ensuring person-centred care.

Regular mental stimulation gives the person with Alzheimer's a feeling of good self-esteem and worth, which we all crave. Even with the short-term-memory loss, it is still worthwhile to see the joy on the faces of the residents after they have accomplished a simple task.

Alzheimer's - Dementia

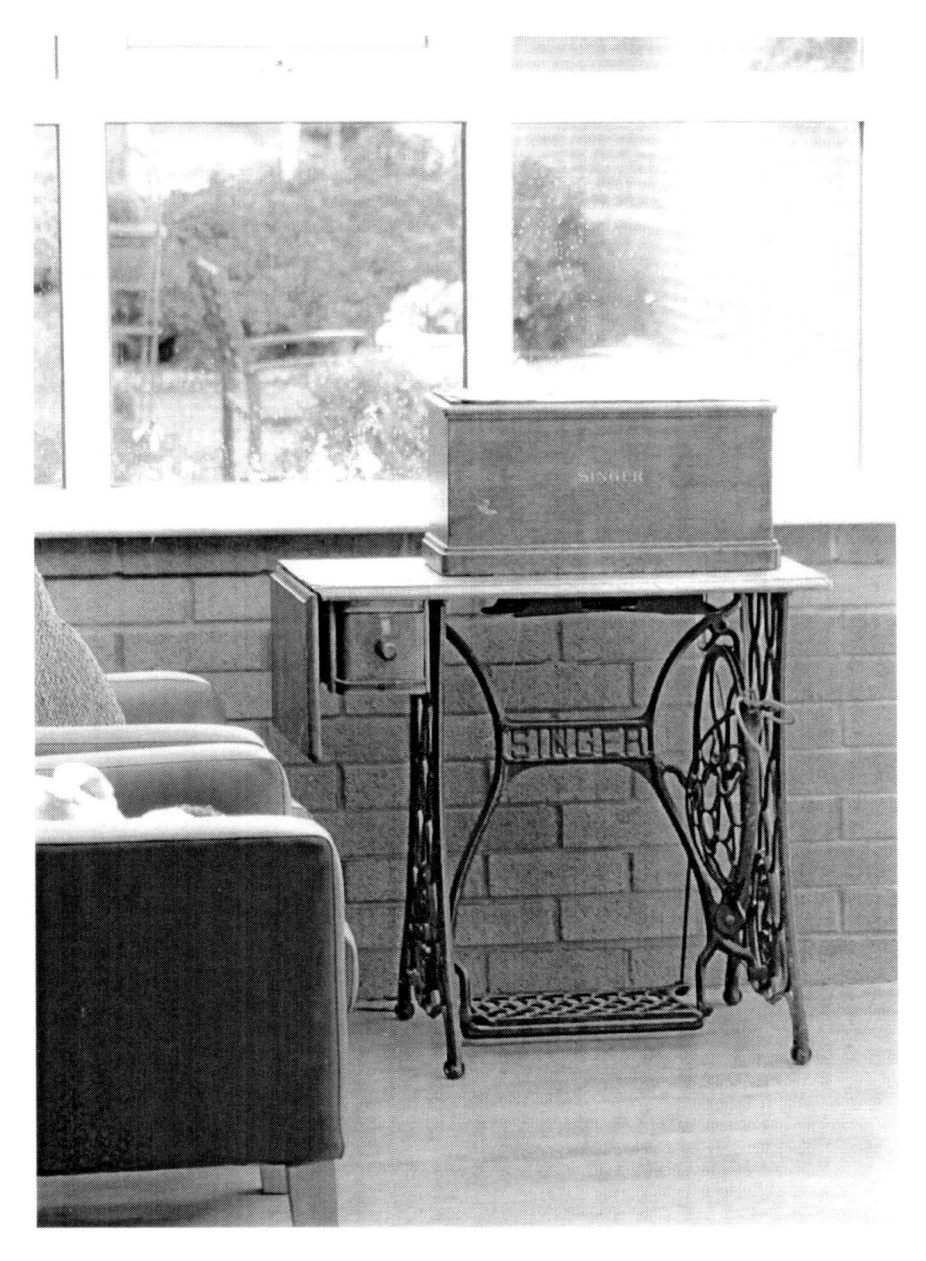

Photograph of a Singer Sewing Machine.

Ann Marie Gallogly

The Singer sewing machine shown in the picture above is a piece of equipment that would have been in a lot of the homes of residents as they were growing up. It didn't need electricity to work, as the foot pedal caused the needle to sew the material. It would have been integral to their everyday life. Its presence in the care home does not just make a great conversation piece for the residents, but it can make the residents feel more at home too.

Music has a great calming effect on everyone in the home, whether it is classical or popular. A piano situated where any resident can play is wonderful therapy for both player and listener. (It is sometimes better if it is an organised music session.)

Alzheimer's - Dementia

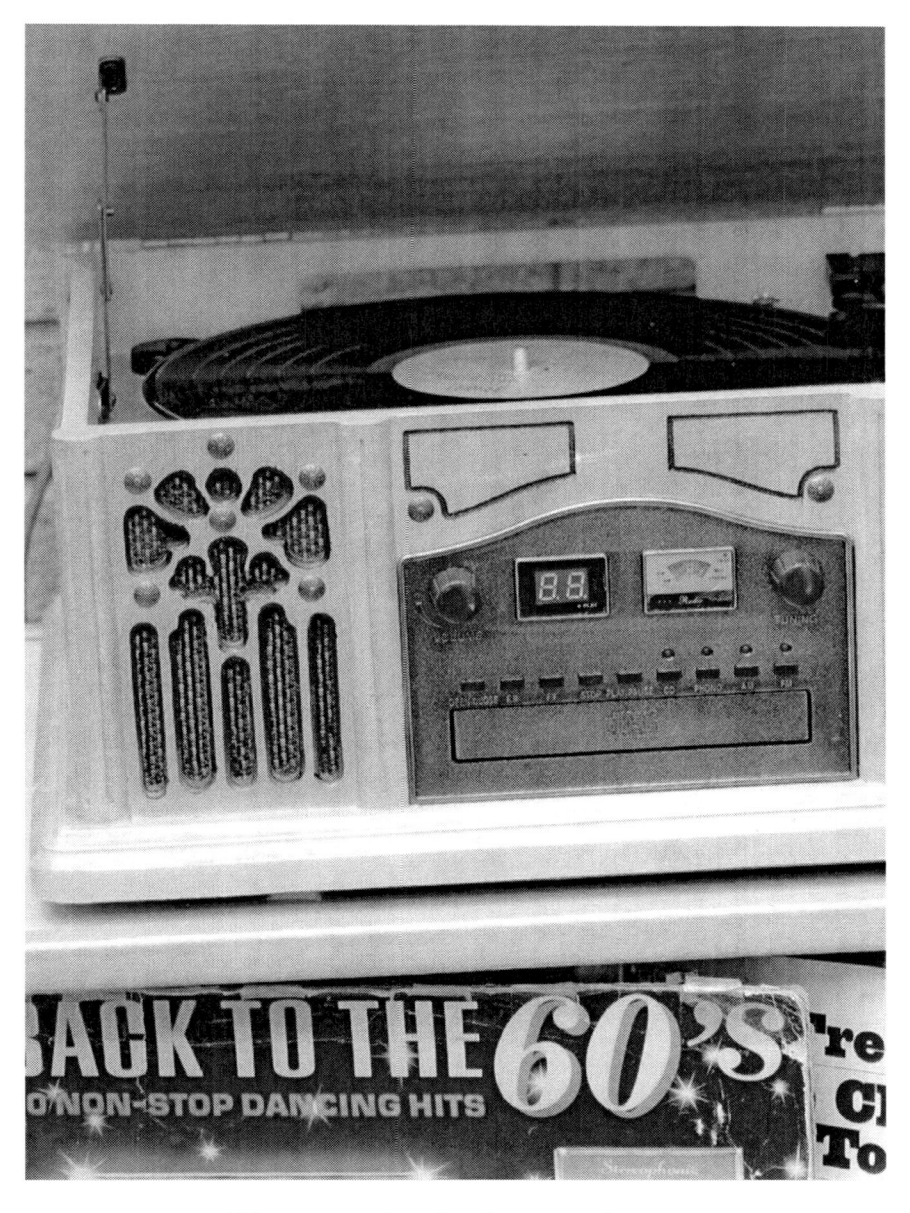

Photograph of a Gramophone.

The old-style record player (gramophone) pictured above and records bring back great memories to those who lived in the 1950s and '60s. The records have the names and pictures of the artists on the cover and the list of songs that are on the record too. A lovely activity for the residents is passing round the record sleeves, talking about the records, and choosing the music they want to listen to. The gramophone was a beautiful piece of equipment that provided entertainment for their families and would have been of great importance to them.

One example below of how an activities person can bring laughter into the residents' lives and remind some residents of their childhood is by taking them to the cinema.

Alzheimer's - Dementia

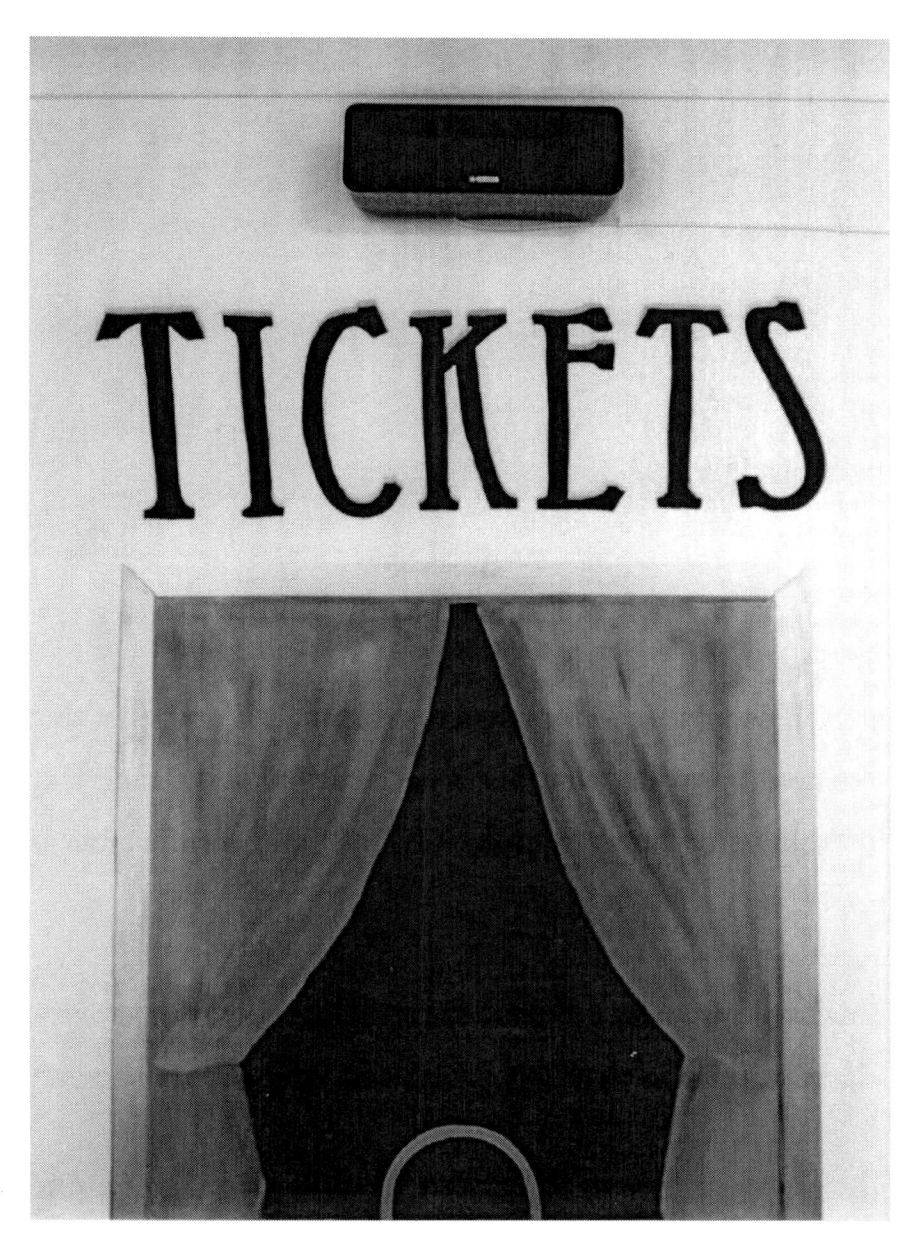

Photograph of Picture of Tickets Kiosk.

Ann Marie Gallogly

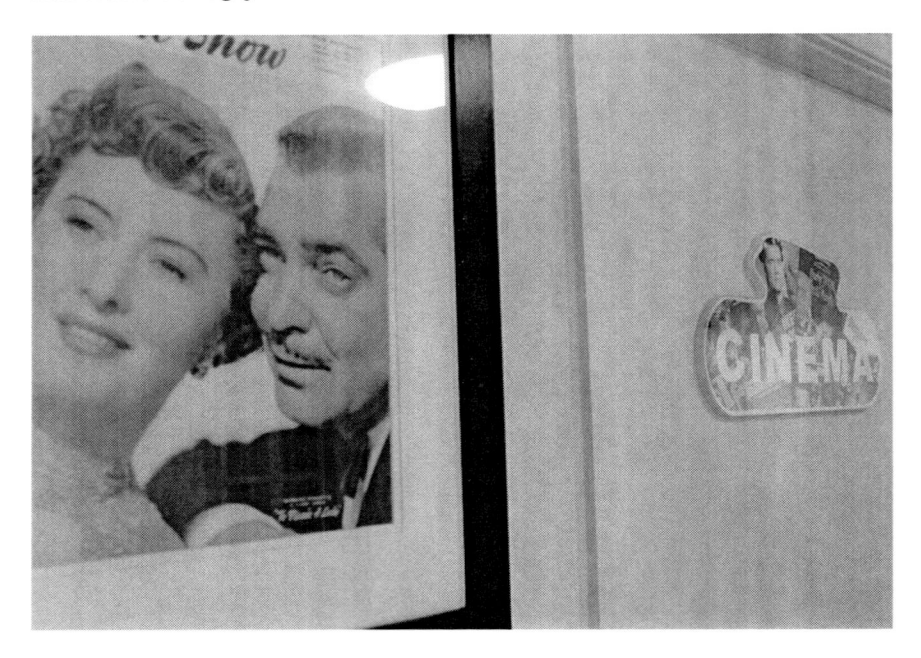

Photograph of Framed picture of Film Stars.

Even if people are ill for whatever reason, it is my belief that we should provide whatever is necessary to make their stay in the nursing home as enjoyable, safe, and comfortable as possible.

This home provides a cinema the residents visit as an activity. Films suitable to their age group and interests are shown.

The above picture of the tickets kiosk is placed to remind residents of 'a trip to the pictures' (as it was known then). This would have been a fond memory.

The picture above, the framed picture of an old film, is placed beside the cinema entrance door. As the residents may recognise the stars of the film, especially Clark Gable, it leaves no doubt about the purpose of the room behind the door.

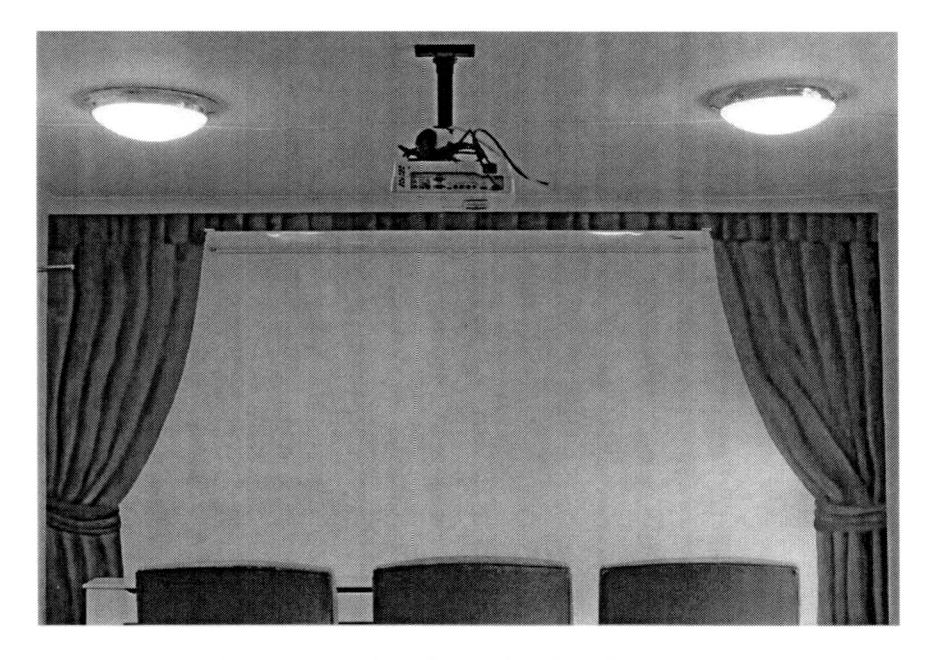

Photograph of inside the Cinema.

Above is a picture of the inside of the cinema. It is designed to try to recreate the residents' past visits to the pictures. The atmosphere in the room, with the heavy curtains pulled closed and pictures of different items of photography, together with the ticket kiosk and the large screen taking up the whole wall, all comes together to make a very pleasant experience that can bring back memories of earlier days, when going to the pictures would have been an enjoyable outing.

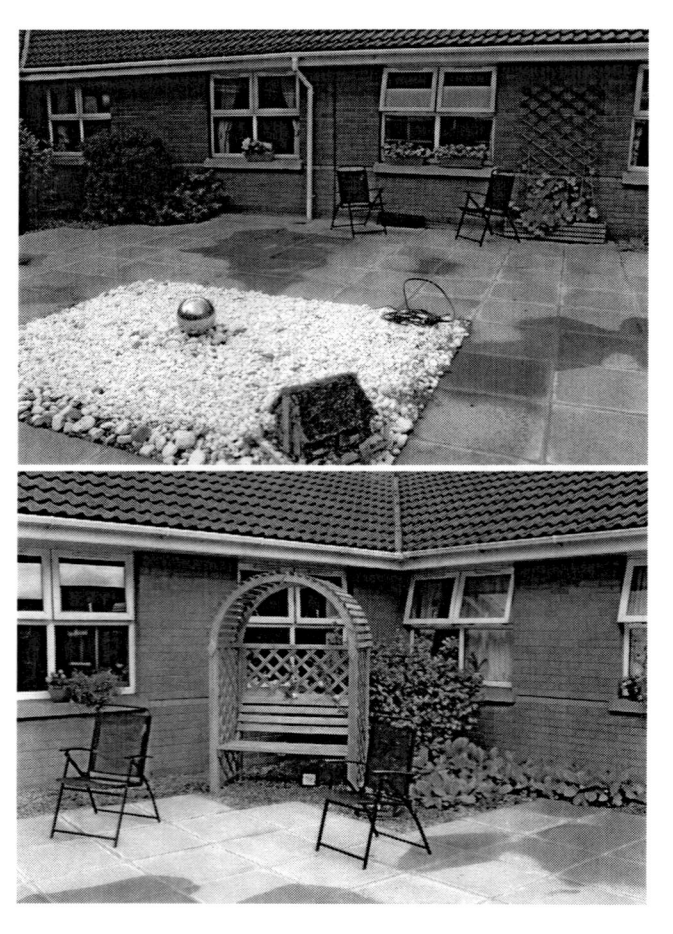

Photograph of Patio.

The patio, which is located within the walls of the home, is easily accessible to the residents, to enter and leave when they wish. Chairs and bench seats are placed so that the residents can sit and enjoy the outdoors and admire the flowers. The activity person provides watering cans for the residents to water the flowers or even weed the plants if needed. This is a lovely place for the residents to sit or walk about freely in a peaceful, safe setting.

Abuse:

I discuss abuse before you visit the home, because this question has worried so many family members. They are often afraid of the unknown, so let's get it dealt with.

Abuse can take many forms; the obvious one that immediately comes to mind is physical abuse. If a resident presents with a bruise or injury to any part of his or her body – for example, a cut or broken bone – the circumstances are investigated in depth by the staff in the home. The injury and cause should be reported, recorded, and attended to as required. It is reported to the doctor, family, and senior home management, who then pass information on to the care management and regulation authorities. Everything is recorded at each stage. If the injury looks suspicious, the authorities investigate and pass on the findings to the appropriate higher legal authorities.

Several possible reasons for the injury come to mind.

A fall due to a wet, slippery floor or a trip hazard can simply be caused by shoelaces not being tied properly. A fall out of bed, being unsteady on their feet, may be due to night-time medication.

Abuse can take the form of verbally chastising a resident who breaks something or who says inappropriate words, speaking to the resident as if he or she is a child. Staff must remember that residents are adults who must be treated with dignity and respect at all times.

It is also abuse if a resident does not get his or her personal hygiene attended to when it is due.

Another form of abuse is restraint, by which a resident is confined to a chair or bed by restraining straps. This is totally illegal, and straps are only advised when someone is being pushed in a wheelchair from one place to another, for example when they cannot walk themselves to the toilet or dining room. Having reached the dining room, the resident is transferred to a soft chair or a chair at a table. If the resident prefers to stay in the wheelchair, that is okay, but waist straps must be freed.

Any form of suspected abuse must be dealt with in the proper manner *immediately.*

Your First Visit to the Home

Walkabout:

It would be a good idea to prepare some questions and take them with you. Make sure to make an appointment, to ensure the manager is available to show you around and answer your questions.

While you are walking around, observe the atmosphere of the home. Does it smell fresh? Can you smell cooking or coffee brewing or flowers or plants? These smells are a positive indicator.

In the morning, the residents should look nice and smell fresh, whether that means being clean-shaven, with aftershave, or perfume. They should be alert looking, with hair combed, dressed nicely, with matching clothes suitable to the weather. (The clothing choice is done purely on what is available in their wardrobe that family have brought in.)

Alzheimer's - Dementia

Be aware if you are visiting after dinner that you will most likely notice some or all of the residents sleeping. This is normal, as the residents are full up after dinner and are only taking a nap. Don't assume it is a drug-induced sleep. You could ask why they are sleeping.

If you are visiting at approximately 4 p.m. onwards, you may notice some residents walking in an aggressive fashion about the corridor. This is what is known as 'sundowning'. This is something that is peculiar to people suffering from Alzheimer's disease.

If your loved one experiences this, you will understand that they are not 'wandering'; they are walking with a purpose. I explain this to my staff, to try to help them with their thoughts. Maybe they want to go home (their childhood home or young-married-life home). Sometimes you may see their partner or a staff member walking with them. This is an excellent sign that everyone knows how to help the person.

First impressions count. For example, not-so-good signs of cleanliness are smells of urine or faeces in open areas, bags of pads sitting about, dirty clothes protectors (bibs used to protect their clothes at mealtimes) sitting about, bins or bags in toilets not emptied, cleaners' trolley left unsupervised with a bag hanging from it full of dirty items, and laundry bags full of clothes not being sent for washing.

A quick indicator of how thoroughly the home is cleaned is gained by taking a quick look at the taps in the lavatories, in particular where the taps join the sink. If this is not cleaned, this is a bad sign of lack of cleanliness.

If you visit at mealtimes, please refer to my article on basic training for new carers serving breakfast, which can be found at the end of part one of this book.

Observe the table setting. For example, are there tablecloths on the tables? Are there salt, pepper, and sauces in the centre? Are the milk jug and sugar bowl empty until the meal starts? If the sugar and milk are put out too early, some of the residents might eat or spill them. Is there a full place setting – cup, saucer, plate, serviettes, knife, fork, dessert spoon, and soup spoon in their correct position?

It is important to have full, complete settings at mealtimes (or it should be ensured the setting is appropriate to the particular diet of the person, the ability of the person to self-feed or not). Maybe the person needs specialized forks and spoons, as he may have difficulty in holding regular cutlery.

This is what I expect a dining room setting to be.

I have seen tables set up with just a cup, plate, and spoon, with no tablecloth. It is undignified.

You may see a carer walking around the corridor with a resident and feeding him at the same time. This is very good practice, as the resident may not sit at the table to eat, so to ensure he gets his full diet, the carer will walk with him, feed him, and assist him.

During your observations, use the senses of sight, smell, touch, and hearing, and especially listen to the sounds of the home. What music is playing? Is it the music of the '60s onwards or the pop music of the present?

After meals, the residents may retire to the sitting room to listen to music or watch television or doze in their armchairs. Not all television programmes for Alzheimer's residents are suitable. They may not recognise or enjoy, for example, *The Simpsons*, but may prefer an old tape that they do recognize, such as Laurel and Hardy. Remember, they are living in the past in their minds. However, current sports programmes may be enjoyable and are a good armchair activity, especially if the resident previously played or supported that sport.

The vacuuming of sitting rooms and washing of floors should be done when the residents are out of that room. Hoovers are very noisy for the residents and can annoy them. Anyone who is likely to get upset with the noise is usually encouraged to go to another area of the home whilst cleaning is being done.

You will see from the following information why the activities therapist can improve the everyday living experience of the residents and a good therapist is invaluable.

Ask whether there is an activities therapist onsite, which is very important in this type of home. One day, a visitor did ask me if she could speak to the therapist, and I asked the therapist if she could oblige. She told me and the visitor of some examples where activities helped the residents. Names are changed for privacy of all, and here are examples of times when activities helped individual residents.

Michael was always working at his shoes. No matter where he was, he was always taking them off and pulling the laces out. Then, of course, the laces and shoes would inevitably get lost or he was walking dangerously around with either one shoe or no laces. After talking to his family about this problem, we discovered he used to work in a shoe factory, making shoes.

Life-stories work, where his life history was obtained, gave a clue as to why he had the problem with his shoes. It was only by speaking to his family that we discovered he used to work in a shoe factory, so he may have had the need for feeling the shoes. Involving Michael in arts and crafts, the therapist gave him lots of various fabrics and textures for him to play with and make collages. This was very stimulating for him, as Michael's behaviour could become very challenging and aggressive. He was a very active man his whole life and played a lot of sport. We made and bought various tactile aids and left them for easy access at all times for Michael and other residents to use. He also loved music, so he was introduced to music therapy, where he would hold and play various musical instruments.

Another resident we will call Annie was chair-bound and required a special chair. None of the staff ever heard her talk. She was always very quiet and subdued until one day our volunteer pet therapist called, and Annie started calling the cat, 'Here, pussy pussy'. We brought the cat over and put it on her lap. She was smiling from ear to ear, stroking and talking to the cat. She obviously was a great lover of cats, and it took her to see and touch one again for us to realise what Annie needed. So we bought her a cat soft toy, and her family brought various cuddly toys to help Annie always feel comfortable and happy at all times. She was never seen again without a furry friend on her lap.

Another resident we will call Mary was a very well-spoken, educated lady and a member of the local music society. She always became very frustrated with staff and fellow residents if their language was not proper or polite.

Ensuring Mary received plenty of stimulation, we always involved her in our music activities. She often talked about playing the piano. At Christmastime, my friend who was a piano teacher came in especially for Mary. We sang carols around the piano whilst my friend played. We asked Mary if she would like to play; she was very happy. She couldn't remember how to play any songs but knew where to place her hands. The piano teacher helped her along, and they chatted about particular songs. We did have an old piano in the care home, and we found that when Mary was sitting beside it, she was always very content and happy. It helped her to engage in conversations with everybody about songs and music. This helped Mary not to become frustrated when trying to think of topics of conversation.

Another resident, John, was a busy farmer his whole life, working on the farm from dawn until dusk when he came to stay with us at the care home. It was very hard for John to sit still for any amount of time. He continuously walked the corridors all day and night. If you asked him where he was going, he'd say he was going home to feed the cows and the sheep. For John to sit still for any amount of time and engage in activities was very short-lived. He would sit for five to ten minutes during our painting class and paint animals, with assistance. During music therapy, he always needed to hold a musical instrument to engage his attention. During spring on my neighbour's farm, one of their lambs required hand-rearing. I asked her if I could take the lamb in to work with me one day especially for John. When John saw the lamb in its little box of hay, he was delighted. He sat down, and I gave him the lamb and its baby bottle of milk, and he fed it. He must have sat for half an hour, caring for and talking to the lamb. It was the most I ever saw him sit still for any amount of time. I tried to engage him at other times with toy animals but to no avail. He always enjoyed pet therapy. He would sit and stroke the dog or cat. On another occasion, we had a rescue sanctuary visit. This was all very stimulating activities for the residents, living in the here and now – living in the moment.

The above stories show that the activity therapist and the care home worked together using reminiscence therapy and life-history work provided by the family of the resident, to give the resident higher self-esteem and a better quality of life.

Further Questions to Ask:

I've heard of rummage boxes. What and where are they? These are boxes or baskets sitting on casual tables with oddments in them for the residents to examine or take away if they wish. A chair is usually beside the table so the resident can sit and browse in comfort. These boxes could include pieces of jewellery, necklaces, bracelets, small magazines, old-style cameras, and photograph albums of local areas of interest that the older generation would recognise.

This shows that the home understands the needs of the Alzheimer's resident to provide stimulation on their own terms.

Ask for evidence and photos of activities that the activities therapist has done and planned for the future.

Is there any evidence of the Alzheimer's Society being involved in the home's activities? They can come into homes and provide weekly music sessions. This is a great source of entertainment for all concerned.

You will likely have a list of questions for the manager. Watch her body language when she is answering your questions. Is she relaxed and willing to show you anything you ask? For example, how does the home provide person-centred care (PCC)? (See university module in part two of this book.)

Is she willing to provide evidence that the home abides by the regulated staffing numbers ratio per resident?

What are the laundry requirements? (Ensure on admission to have all the resident's clothes name-tagged or marked with marker pen.)

Everyone knows how socks get eaten up in the washing at home. Imagine all the clothes unmarked in a nursing home; it does not bear thinking about. The risk of losing clothes is well increased if not marked. Unique identifying initials on the clothes label are enough.

You could ask the manager about staff training, for example to explain COSHE (Control of Substances Hazardous to Environment) for example, cleaning liquids, moving and handling, challenging behaviour, abuse, and any training done by the Alzheimer's Society in the home. Her answers will indicate the quality of care to be provided by fully trained staff of all levels.

Observe whether the manager is friendly to all the residents you meet on the walkabout and whether she calls them by their names. This is an excellent indicator, as previously one of my visitors explained why she chose my home above others she viewed. She said it was highly recommended by a friend, and she saw for herself when she first viewed that the manager spoke to everyone by their first name.

Observe the staff when they are working with the residents. Are they speaking to them in a dignified manner? Some residents like to be spoken to in first-name terms and others by their title, such as Mister, Missus, Doctor, or Judge, and this is ascertained at admission by them and their family.

The manager should be asked how they deal with challenging behaviour. What is it? Does the nurse automatically give them drugs to sedate them?

This is a big worry for the family. Challenging behaviour occurs when the resident hits out at staff or other residents. Remember, these other residents are vulnerable adults too.

There are various reasons for this behaviour. I will talk more about that further on.

The appropriate way for the above incident to be managed would be to gently remove Joe and any stressed residents from the situation, make everyone a cup of tea, and introduce an activity that suits the residents concerned, to help everyone move on and redirect their thoughts.

Drugs should not be the first protocol; medication is never given by the nurse unless it is ordered by the doctors.

If you witness challenging behaviour during your visit, this is good. Do not be scared; it is an opportunity to see how the staff handle the situation, and it should reassure you on how your loved one will be treated in your absence.

Some More Questions to Ask the Manager:

One of the most frequently asked questions is, can we personalise the room? This could involve bringing in pictures and paintings from home.

This is a wonderful idea for the resident. Sometimes the family brings in their own bedclothes like duvet covers, throws, cushions, etc. Of course the home supplies these items, but it makes the room more familiar to residents when they see their own items.

One word of caution here: it is a better idea to have pictures that hang on the wall rather than ones that sit on the dressing table, especially if it is a special photo or picture. A picture with regular glass might get dropped and broken, so for safety reasons, hanging pictures might be better.

I do advise families not to bring in original special photos, as the resident may lift the photograph and leave it in another room or even put it in a bag which may get disposed of. If you really want to put photos or other items on the dressing table, copy them and put them in a safe frame to place on the dressing table. If it gets mislaid, then no harm done, as you can always recopy the photograph from the original.

An even better idea, which is safer again, is to photocopy a special photo and get it laminated. This means the resident can carry the photo about with her; there is no glass to cause injury, and it can be easily cleaned. It won't get torn or ripped up either. If it gets lost, another can be laminated, and the resident is happy looking at her favourite photo. You then know your loved one is happy viewing this photo in your absence, which also gives you some consolation and reassurance.

You and your loved one will feel more relaxed in a room filled with loving memories in a safe environment.

Ask the manager about the home's policy on jewellery. Everyone loves their own jewellery, and you can take it into the home for your loved one to wear, but again use caution and common sense. The major problem with Alzheimer's sufferers is their short-term memory loss, and if the family heirloom went missing, it would be such a shame.

Copies can be made of the most expensive items and the copy brought in with your loved one. They will be just as happy with the copies, and you will not be so worried if they do go missing.

Insurance policies may not pay out for lost items by an Alzheimer's resident in a care home. If the original was lost, the sentimental and financial loss would only add to the other worries you already have.

A special word about reading glasses, which residents can easily remove themselves: these can also be personalised, either by getting the optician to imprint the name on the frame or doing it yourself. I have, on occasion, with the family's permission, had to paint a little nail varnish onto the frame to identify similar glasses. The colour of nail varnish was recorded into the care plan of each resident and easily found when a problem situation arose.

The same problem can arise with dentures, and these too can be personalised by the dentist. If the resident has lost his teeth or is even wearing the wrong ones (this can happen but very seldom does), this can affect eating, therefore affecting food intake and causing weight loss.

Weight Loss:

How do you monitor Joe if he loses weight? He should be weighed upon admission and weekly if he loses weight after a month or if he is not eating his meals. The dietician will be brought in and food supplements ordered, and he will be put on a food and weight chart.

How do you monitor if your loved one won't sit on the weighing scales and is unable to stand? Inform him that you are going to weigh him and afterward that he is going to have his meal.

The technique I use is to place the weighing chair at the table and encourage the resident to sit at the table for his meal. This may take a few attempts, as the chair is large and slippery, in other words different from dining room chairs.

Set the scales at the weight that he was at the last weigh-in, and as soon as he sits on the chair, weigh him. Thus the weight is recorded.

It is very important to ensure that regular weight recordings are taken, so the dietician can recommend the correct supplement, especially if the resident has continually been losing weight. He should be on a food chart, where a record is kept of the amount of the meal actually eaten. This will show if he does not eat certain foods or is refusing his food for other reasons.

Pain:

How do you monitor Joe if he has pain? Does pain show up as challenging behaviour? Yes, sometimes a person suffering from Alzheimer's will show challenging behaviour simply by shouting or hitting out, as he doesn't know how else to express his physical pain. This is where the trained staff use their professional judgement to act accordingly.

Elderly people experience pain, whether they have Alzheimer's disease or not. Many have problems with constipation, so a daily laxative if ordered by the doctor would alleviate this problem. Maybe they have arthritis and the pain in the bones is a constant cause of discomfort; a mild painkiller may solve this problem. Many elderly people do complain of pain in the bones, especially someone who can't change position in a chair or bed. An electric ripple cushion or mattress, which automatically moves the ripples underneath the person and so relieves the cause of the pressure by constantly alternating the ripples, will solve that problem.

I am mentioning pain here, as I have a great fear of pain myself, and I would like you to know how it would be assessed in someone with Alzheimer's. We all know that people with Alzheimer's have great difficulty expressing themselves, so how do we assess and diagnose the cause of their pain and treat it? It is difficult to get a straight answer to the question 'Have you any pain?' Each home has a pain-assessment tool to help answer the question, and with the help of body language, gestures, and past history, it may indicate where and how intense the pain is.

Body language can sometimes be difficult to ascertain, but by knowing the resident and the physical symptoms, an assessment is made. Joe may say he has a sore foot, and by examining his foot for any injury to either foot or toes, a decision is made as to whether anything abnormal is found. If nothing abnormal is found, then it is more likely that his stomach ulcer is playing up, as he has a history of it. Pain is pain, no matter where, and must be treated with appropriate medication and a record kept to see if it is relieved.

The doctor is informed and examines Joe, diagnosing the cause and prescribing pain relief. The nurse administers this and records the effect of pain relief. If Joe is still experiencing pain, as with any person suffering, the problem would need further investigation. It may be necessary to admit Joe to hospital, and the nurse will send a transfer letter with Joe including particulars and instructions on how to communicate with him.

Challenging Behaviour/ Distress Reaction:
Challenging behaviour is otherwise known as distressed reaction.

What is challenging behaviour? Does the nurse automatically give drugs to sedate the resident? These are some of the questions families worry and ask about.

As the name implies, it is a reaction to a situation in which the resident does not know how to show his or her distress, except by verbally or physically lashing out. This reaction may be caused by discomfort, the result of pain, fear of people, or their surroundings or whatever moment they are living in.

I have addressed challenging behaviour briefly within the section 'Your First Visit to the Home'. Within the care environment, it is a sign that something is wrong and needs to be rectified, possibly a need of the resident not being met or a problem with communication. The challenging behaviour, if not sorted, can lead to verbal or physical abuse by the resident.

People suffering from Alzheimer's forget the words for everyday simple things. They make up words or even try to say something using parts of words. Staff are familiar with the resident and come to recognise what it is the person is trying to say. They may say yes but really mean no, and when the item offered is wrong, they will get cross if it is the wrong interpretation. Then challenging behaviour presents, but we now know the cause and can deal with it.

Are there other causes for challenging behaviour? Yes, certainly there are. Noise, for example, the vacuum cleaner or too many people talking at the one time.

The person gets distressed when he can't express his feelings or thoughts to you, when someone invades her space, when someone sits on *his* chair in the dining room or sitting room, when she wants to go to the toilet but can't get up by herself to go, when he wants to go to bed but can't say so, or when she is feeling thirsty but unable to express it.

There are many reasons for this behaviour, and the more we know about a new resident on admission, the less likely the new resident will show challenging behaviour. With the help of the family, the staff can get a full picture of the resident's likes, dislikes, food preferences, bedtime routines, and any information the family needs to tell us, especially if it is something as simple as informing us that we should not put milk in his tea, as he normally takes it black.

Below are further examples of why the resident may show challenging behaviour.

Looking for a Start:

Jack would awaken as early as 6 a.m., get dressed, and come to staff and say, 'I'm looking for a start.' He got really angry when we did not understand what he meant. Challenging behaviour continued all day as he kept repeating 'I'm looking for a start.' We contacted the family, and they were able to explain what this meant. As Jack had worked in the construction industry, he had to go out to look for work. He went to a new building site at 6 a.m. and stood in line outside the foreman's site hut and said to the foreman,

'I'm looking for a start.' This meant he was available and willing to work.

This was recorded, and all staff were informed, especially the night staff. The family recommended that we ask Jack his name and his trade, write it down, and tell him work on site starts tomorrow. This is what the site foreman would have done and said. This simple procedure satisfied Jack, and he continued on his normal activities for the remainder of the day. No challenging behaviour was caused as a result of the staff not knowing what he was talking about.

Young staff or overseas staff would not be expected to know old local sayings or their meanings, but these sayings are well known by older members of society where we live. The senior staff are invaluable in helping to translate the sayings and explaining to the staff on duty these meanings. The saying and meaning is entered into the resident's care plan, and then every member of staff is informed.

Spend a Penny:

Another local saying comes to mind and is frequently used by residents in the area: 'I want to spend a penny.' Years ago, to gain access and use a public toilet, a penny coin was put in the slot in the door to open it. So to spend a penny means 'I want to go to the toilet.' It is very obvious why challenging behaviour would be presented when a resident is not understood and cannot get to the toilet.

Money Issues:

Another issue may be money problems. Not having cash is a big problem for some residents, especially as money can get lost or thrown away or hidden very easily. One resident in particular, 'Jack', got very distressed and presented with challenging behaviour when he had no money in his wallet. His family did give him some cash when they visited, but he was forever losing it or hiding it, and the family could not afford to keep giving more and more, especially as there was nowhere for him to spend it, as all his requirements were provided for him.

While discussing the problem with Jack, he explained that he was not getting paid for his week's work. Jack had worked in the construction industry all his adult life and got paid in cash in an envelope on Fridays. He was feeling undervalued, as he was not getting paid for working all week and got cross and anxious, especially on Fridays or whatever day he thought was Friday.

His family was very distressed too and dreaded visiting Jack, so they asked me for help. We discussed this, and at the end, we decided to photocopy paper money from the former currency available during Jack's working life. We got suitable paper, photocopied both sides, and cut around the edges. We crinkled the notes to make them look used and put them in an envelope with Jack's name on it. He was delighted to get his pay packet again, and his family was relieved that Jack was feeling of value again. This also solved the family's money worries, as when Jack needed more 'money', more was photocopied and put aside for the next Friday.

This was a very unconventional procedure, but it does show the extra step a good home is willing to make to ensure that the resident feels valued, also allowing the family to feel more relaxed and happy. This is all done with the permission of the home manager and above all, done for the good of the resident.

As a direct result of intervention, Jack's body language changed immediately and considerably. He walked straighter, with a confident swagger and purpose. He smiled and talked to everyone who would listen. It was a delight to see, especially as it solved that challenging behaviour, as he felt he had his dignity and self-respect back.

This is a great example of the importance of getting a full record of a resident's life history, including his work and hobbies. This helps us to determine potential causes of challenging behaviour. We can then work on the answer with the resident and his family's input.

Day-/Night-Time Routines:

The first night the resident is admitted, the carer should refer to the care plan and the sleep patterns as described by the family. It may say that he likes to retire about 8 p.m., wears bed socks and pyjama trousers or maybe long johns (some men don't wear pyjama trousers in bed, only underpants), sleeps with two pillows and an incontinence aid (pad). At home, he is helped to get up from 8 a.m. onwards.

This can be a very unsettling time for those experiencing Alzheimer's disease. Preparation and routine are very important. Staff need to ensure Joe eats a good supper, is assisted to change for bed, and is settled in his own room. Some residents, after taking their night medication as prescribed by their doctor, like to watch television, read a book of choice, or listen to music.

However, Joe finds it very difficult to relax; sometimes he continually walks around the unit, and/or bangs his hands on the walls. He never speaks to anyone, and this can go on until the early hours of the morning.

Then one night, I took Joe by the hand and walked with him to his room. I suggested to him that he lie on top of the bed. He did, and he looked at me with big, sad eyes and never spoke. I then proceeded to say 'Shuuuush' quietly. Joe made to get up, and I loudly repeated 'Shuuush'. Joe lay back down on his bed. I slowly walked away from him towards the door, continuing to say 'Shuuush' quietly. I sat at the open bedroom door where Joe could watch me, making my voice lower – 'Shuuush', then lower again, and lo and behold, Joe fell asleep. I then continued with my other duties of the night. This gentleman was about fifty-five years of age and came from a professional musical background.

Joe slept all night. The sound of a childhood 'shuuush' and the company reassured Joe, and he felt safe.

This is one example of the special needs of the individual and is learnt by the staff when they know the needs of the person (PCC – person-centred care). This was the right technique for Joe. Finding the right technique for each resident is very rewarding for all.

A reason for a resident's challenging behaviour may be a result of refusing his medication. This would be recorded and his own doctor informed. The doctor may refer the resident back to the consultant, who will review his medication.

The family may, at these times, be contacted, and they will come into the home to help defuse the situation. This may help the resident, who is feeling distressed and may respond better to his own family.

Drugs should not be the first protocol; medication is *never* given by the nurses unless it is ordered by the doctor.

Ann Marie Gallogly

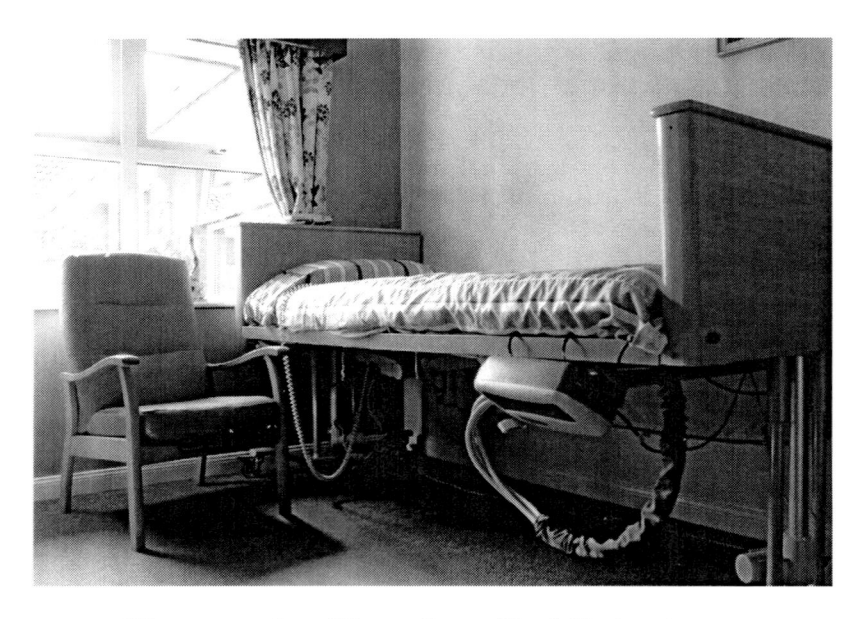

Photograph of Low Low Bed Raised.

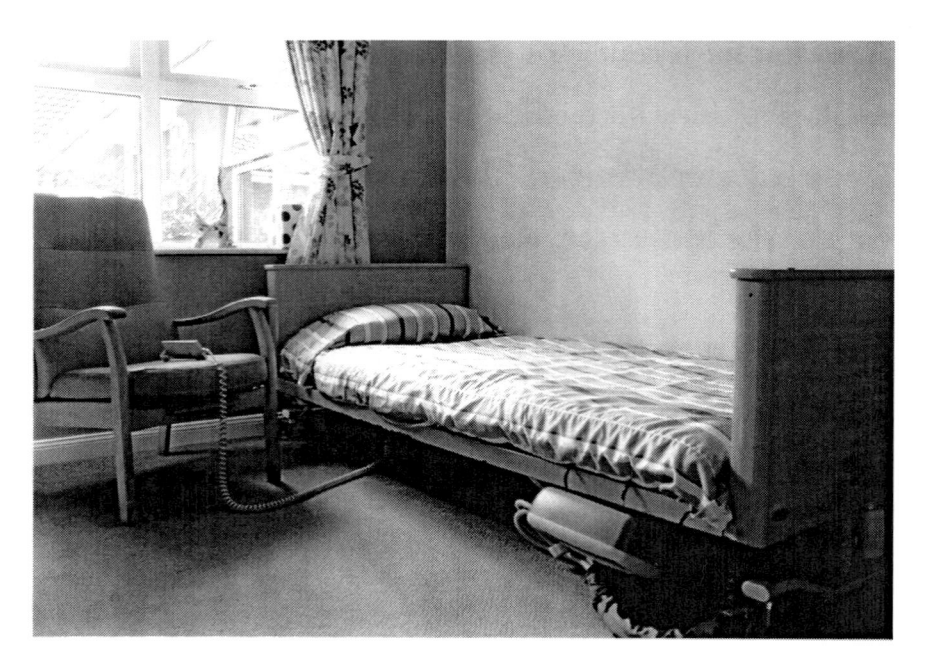

Photograph of Low Low Bed Lowered.

Alzheimer's - Dementia

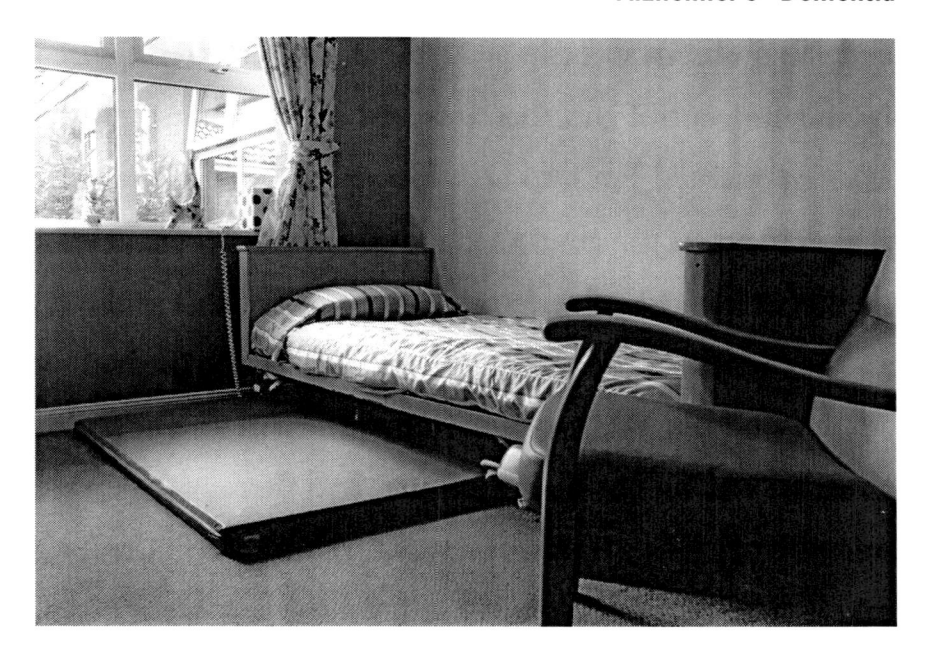

Photograph of Low Low Bed Lowered
with Mattress on Floor.

The three pictures above all show a type of bed used in the homes called a 'low low bed' in its two positions, up and down and with a mattress placed beside the bed. The case study below explains its need.

Another resident we'll call Jim was forever falling out of bed, as he was very restless in his sleep, and he was in great danger of seriously hurting himself. Bed rails were not suitable, as Jim could climb over them, at a greater risk of injury. A new type of bed was purchased for him, a low low bed. This was an electric bed, frame, and mattress, raised by remote control and then lowered almost to the ground after we assisted Jim into bed. However, this did not solve the problem, as Jim continued to roll out of bed, but at least he was at less risk of serious injury. To solve this problem, another mattress was placed on the floor beside the bed for Jim to land on. We had a movement alarm that sounded when he was on the floor mattress, and therefore we were immediately able to ensure he was comfortable on the floor mattress, so he could sleep soundly for the rest of the night.

This is not a common practice, to nurse people on the floor, but we try to provide person-centred care (PCC) for each individual when the resident presents with a challenge. Jim was treated with dignity, respect, and privacy at all stages of the procedure.

On reading Jim's history from social workers, it indicated that Jim had lived a rough life on the streets for many years, so maybe he felt more comfortable on the floor for this reason.

There are many reasons for challenging behaviour, based on the person's own history, whether it be at night or during the day. The following story is a very common example.

I've Lost My Baby:

A little lady of eighty-six years of age started to show challenging behaviour in the afternoons. By this I mean she would walk and even run along the corridor (sundowning), and believe me she was very fit. When trying to find the cause of this sudden behaviour, I asked Rose where she was going. She kept saying, 'I've lost my baby.' Her family loved her very much, but due to her Alzheimer's disease, she could not be cared for at home for various reasons. Every mother knows that feeling of pure panic if her child should disappear, in a shopping centre for example, even if it is only for a minute. This was the feeling Rose had when she was running about the home.

I discussed the situation with the family, and we agreed to introduce a doll and cradle into her room. Would you believe it – this doll gave Rose so much comfort, especially in the afternoons. Rose would walk quietly around the corridor nursing her baby when she needed that feeling of giving and receiving love.

This example again shows the importance of knowing family history and the personality of resident in her younger life, even though the resident may have changed after Alzheimer's disease affected her.

Mealtime Dos and Don'ts:

I've included a sample of the instructions I give new carers, especially overseas staff, on the dining room experience. The new carer should be partnered with an experienced carer. Obviously, more formal training is given later.

Basic Training for New Carers or Nursing Assistants Serving Breakfast

Do say good morning to each resident at the table. As you are assisting someone to that table, say, 'Good morning, Joe; good morning, Sarah, etc.' Don't forget to talk to the residents. Make each meal a pleasant occasion, and sit at the table beside them.

Don't stand while assisting the resident to eat or drink.

Alzheimer's - Dementia

Do get to know the residents' likes, dislikes, special diet, allergies, and seating positions.

Do assist the residents at their usual place at the table, as they like to sit at the same place every mealtime.

Do make sure they are sitting beside someone they like.

Don't place them beside someone who will annoy them; gently remove someone who has sat in the wrong seat. Ask for assistance from another member of staff if necessary.

Do ensure that the wheelchair footrests are moved back and the waist straps are unlocked while the resident is sitting at the table.

Do ask the resident if he would like a clothes protector on, and proceed to put it on him if accepted.

Don't just wrap it around him and not explain what you are doing.

Do pour the orange juice into the glass and then proceed to pour the milk into the teacups.

Don't ever pour hot tea into a teacup without **first** putting in the milk.

Don't fill the cup too full, as it could spill; they can always get more.

Do make sure that that any resident who is allergic to regular milk gets the appropriate milk, for example soya milk.

Do ask them if they want sugar; some residents can take their own sugar, so place the sugar beside them to help themselves.

Don't put sugar into the cup of a resident who is diabetic; know all special diets.

The kitchen staff will serve out the porridge.

Do ask the resident if they want porridge or cornflakes or whatever they want; then place it in front of them.

Do assist them if they want milk and sugar in the porridge; make sure the spoon is beside the bowl. While they are all eating the porridge, proceed to pour the tea.

Do ensure the cup is on their right side (if they are right-handed), close to their reach.

Don't pour the tea from the left side (if they are right-handed), as this would mean the teapot being directly in front of their body whilst pouring.

Don't reach across the table to pour tea always ensure to stand beside the resident.

Don't place the hot teapot on the top of the breakfast trolley; put it on the lower shelf, just in case a resident decides to help himself. *Never* place it anywhere else, for example the breakfast table.

Do give out the toast for anyone who wants it, and open the marmalade, as the packets are hard to open, especially if the resident has arthritis.

Do let them put the marmalade on the toast themselves, and only do it for them if they ask or are unable to do it for themselves. Place the toast on the left side, close to the resident. Some residents are short-sighted and may not be able to see their plate.

Do fill out a food and fluid balance intake chart to record their food intake.

Do observe that the resident has actually eaten his or her food. If not, ask why, and ask if the resident wants something different to eat.

Don't just lift the plate and not observe that the meal was fully eaten; if not, record it on the resident's food chart and note if this is a regular occurrence. Check if the resident is losing weight; if so, this may be the reason. Record and report any worries to the nurse in charge.

Benefits of the Care/Nursing Home

Now that you are informed of some of the things that can present a challenge in a nursing care environment, you may still be worrying – but now you are an informed person. Let's look at the benefits for you and your loved one after arriving in this new environment.

The Alzheimer's home is a home away from home, in a secure, safe setting, with code locks to prevent anyone walking out into the outside world, where they may get lost. In their own home, was this a big worry? Yes.

Within the nursing home, the resident will be able to walk around safely, in a building that has been built or developed for that purpose, which gives the resident some freedom.

Professionally trained staff are present to provide for their personal care 24/7, including activities for their mental stimulation. There is input from outside services such as tissue-viability specialists, occupational therapists, dieticians, dental services, and optical services, to name a few, all overseen by staff nurses and managers who develop care plans with your help and continued input.

The whole building and the services provided are inspected by the government authority, and if it does not conform to the regulations, the home may even be closed down. Staff are regulated and police checked to make sure they are suitable to work with vulnerable adults.

Your loved one is never lonely, with all the activities provided, and his needs are assessed regularly, with you visiting when you wish.

It is sometimes hard for the family to come to terms with their loved one growing an attachment with the staff. This is normal and good for the resident; he knows he is well cared for. Even if he cannot express it in words, he will in body language.

You will know whether you have made a good decision when you see the standard of care in the home, and your life can move on too, alongside that of your loved one.

Even if your loved one's physical and mental abilities deteriorate, you know you should be kept informed, and with the knowledge and faith in the care home, you will both be able to face the future together. You are not alone.

Information Is Priceless

Choosing the right nursing home for your family should enrich your loved one's life experience in the face of adversity and also give you peace of mind.

It is very important to understand that you can always call unannounced, to view the home again when the manager is not there, to confirm your decision. See for yourself if all the questions you asked are answered by the evidence you see. You are informed now and can make an informed decision.

A few words on families' guilt: Your loved one, in the past, may have indicated an unwillingness to be put in a residential or nursing home. How do you get over the family guilt about placing them in a home?

The resident may want to go home, but to what home? Is she looking to go home to her parents' house? The family home that she built and where she reared her family? Or whatever part of her life that she felt safe and secure in?

What area of the memory is your loved one in?

This is where the different areas of training given should show when staff can help the person through with activities by diverting his or her thoughts somewhere else.

When they expressed a desire not to be put in a home, they might not have known what they were asking of their family or the extent to which their personality and life would change because of this disease. If the person has previously said he would never wish to go into a care home, this wish may well have been expressed when he was in full health, and he did not know how the effects of Alzheimer's would change his life. The quality of life in the care home versus living at home must be seen to improve his safety, mental stimulation, physical well-being, and just as important, the physical and mental health of his carers and family.

My Mother

Finally, we come to my own personal experience. I have been discussing so far the nurse's point of view on how a resident should be cared for in a nursing/care home. I am going to share with you my family's thoughts, feelings, and fears when I was the daughter of a resident, whilst I was also her nurse and she was a resident in the home where I worked.

My mother spent the last four years of her life in the nursing home. Circumstances ruled that she couldn't be cared for at her home, and it was a major decision for me, my brother, and sisters.

She settled in well, enjoyed her food, and was happy to accept all care and attention given. She took part in activities. Unfortunately, she did not initiate conversations with others, but she would answer when spoken to or when a question was asked.

She watched me working on the floor, for example, doing medications. I chose not to do her personal care, and that was okay too.

After she was admitted, we took her shopping for new clothes. She was smiling and picked the clothes herself, the colour and style she liked. Her whole demeanour changed after a short while in the home. She sat up more confidently and smiled more often. My family were very happy for her and us.

I have heard relatives express that their loved one did not know them, and they were very upset by this. I tell them the story of the day I went to visit Mother wearing my ordinary clothes, not my nurse's uniform. I entered the sitting room and pulled a chair over beside her. I greeted her and said to the man beside her, 'Hello, James. How are you?' Next thing I knew, Mother put her hand onto my knee and said 'You are *my* visitor.' I was speechless that she actually recognised me as someone special – *I was hers.* It was the first time I realised this, and I was very happy for that small blessing. She had never called me her daughter, so I was not aware of who she thought I was. It didn't matter in the end, as long as she thought *I was her visitor*, someone special.

My family felt the best option for my mother was to be admitted into the home that I was working in, because there was a bed available, because of the location, because of the good reputation of the home, and especially because I worked there. It was with a certain amount of fear that I agreed, as I wasn't sure how other staff, residents, and their families – and more importantly, Mother herself – would accept it. My mother was very happy there for the remainder of her days, with her special visitors. The staff and other visitors saw for themselves that I gave the same care and attention to their loved one as I gave to Mother. I told my family if they had any concerns about Mother's care to give it first to Mother's primary nurse, not me. This was the only way I could cope.

The primary nurse is allocated to each resident upon admission. It is she who is responsible for writing her care plan and instructing other staff on how to nurse the resident. She liaises with outside professionals when necessary and is responsible for seeing that her instructions are carried out. The family should inform her of any concerns or any new information they need to tell us.

Mother and her special visitors settled into a happy relationship with the support of staff and other families.

Nursing in Pre-Private-Nursing-Home Times

Way back in the 1970s, I worked night duty in a typical care home setting of the time, wherein the 'patients' were nursed in large, open wards with about thirty beds in each and only one bathroom and toilet attached. The only privacy was a mobile curtained screen that was rolled to each bed when the nurse was performing nursing aid. The patients sat on a soft chair beside the bed with a trolley table in front of them for the purpose of eating their meals or placing drinks on.

To give you a feel for what it was like back then, I'll tell you a story of an incident that occurred during night duty. Around three o'clock in the morning, a man about eighty years of age called out, 'Nurse', and he explained that he could not pass urine while lying in bed. I assisted him to the toilet, where he still could not do it, so I turned on the water taps in the sink and the bath. The sound of running water helps people to urinate, especially when having difficulty. It worked, and the man went back to bed happy and comfortable.

Now what I did not think of was, it was three o'clock in the morning, the ward was very quiet, and sound travels. The sound of all those taps running had travelled into the ward, and all the patients heard it. How did I know that? At 6 a.m., when I was checking the patients' beds as we did every morning to ensure they were dry and comfortable, *all* the beds were wet, and I had to change everyone before day staff came on duty at 8 a.m.

There was absolutely no privacy or dignity in the old regimen of nursing care. For that reason alone, I thank God for private nursing homes with the single bedrooms and toilet facilities within.

Testimonials

I work in the same home as Sister Ann, who is a professional, caring, and understanding nurse. These qualities are shown in her ability to be a team leader who is also a part of that team.

She keeps up to date with all training and ensures we do too. With her excellent communication skills and understanding of new starts and overseas staff in their problems, she ensures to give us support to give the best care to the residents, who come first, always.

Joan Magin, Northern Ireland, Senior Care Assistant.

An efficient nurse as well as a sister, who works on the floor with us. She encouraged me when she was my mentor when I first worked with her four years ago She taught me dementia care, and I thank God for having Sister Ann as my mentor.

Celine Kurian, RGN, India.

In October 2004 I left from Singapore for Northern Ireland. I had worked as a private nurse for the late Prime Minister and was recruited to work in UK as a senior carer in one of the care homes. Ann Gallogly, a registered nurse in her profession, was the sister in charge on our floor She was very eloquent and cogent. Sister Ann was always there to reassure and guide me in the workplace.

Thank you Sr Ann for the encouragement you gave me so that I enhanced my skills and knowledge. I won't forget you.

Maria Nimfa Magbanua. Essex. UK.

My opinion as a Deputy Manager having worked as a Registered Nurse Alongside Sister Ann on the same unit, I have found her to be extremely competent in her role.

She has great rapport with the residents and also with their loved ones. She excels at communication skills. Families are always advised in the first instance of any changes to their loved ones status.

Jean Heatley RGN Deputy Manager. N Ireland.

I worked as an Activities Therapist in a Care Centre in Newry alongside Ann Gallogly for Five years organising activities for individuals and groups of older people with Alzheimer's and Dementia. I found her very professional and totally committed to ensuring that the safety and welfare of the residents was kept to a high standard at all times.

Caroline Shimmons,
Activities Therapist, Northern Ireland.

Part 2

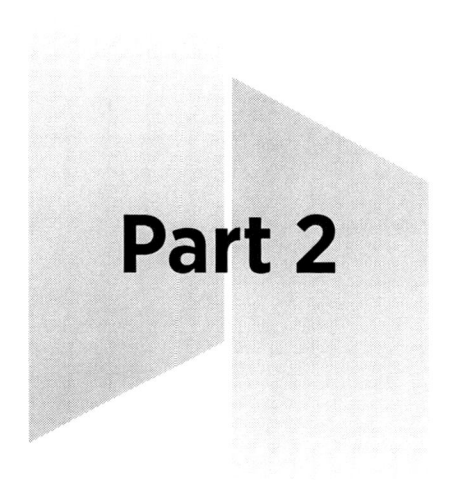

This part of my information guide includes excerpts from my university module on the history of dementia and what person-centred care means and how it improves the life of the person with Alzheimer's disease.

A History of Dementia

In order to discuss the 'inevitable decline' referred to in this question, the author will demonstrate why it may have been inevitable in the past for people to decline and die from dementia, but with current care, funding, treatment, research, and knowledge, it seems now that it is not so simple as an inevitable decline into dependency (Cheston and Bender 2003).

According to the International Classification of Diseases (ICD 10 2002), dementia is defined as 'A syndrome due to disease of the brain, usually of a chronic or progressive nature in which there is disturbance of multiple higher cortical function including memory, thinking, orientation, comprehension, calculation, learning capability, language and judgement. Consciousness is not impaired. Impairments of cognitive function are commonly accompanied, occasionally preceded, by deterioration in emotional control, social behaviour or motivation.'

The author would be of the opinion that historically, people with dementia have suffered as a result of a poor awareness and understanding from the public, combined with the stigma associated with both mental illness and old age. In the past, patients were admitted to institutions (insane asylums), away from public view, with little or no privacy, dignity, stimulation, or family input (Goffman 1963). These institutions had large dormitories for patients and lacked in social, recreational, and bathing facilities. They had very under-resourced wards and little medical provision, except for doctors seeing patients with physical illness or signing death certificates (Jolley and Arie 1978, as cited in Marshall 2005). The aforementioned reflects the author's family experiences of dementia care.

In the 1970s, when the author was a student nurse, the words 'pre-senile dementia' or 'senile' were used to describe patients experiencing the illness. Research from Fox (1989) showed that 'senile dementia' was the fourth-leading cause of death in the United States. Katzman and Karasu (as cited in Fields 1975) suggested that establishing dementia as an illness with a high mortality rate rather than an aspect of ageing would aid attempts at greater funding. This made dementia more acceptable to the public, as the stigma (Goffman 1963) of mental disease was reduced, and research might find a cure.

In Northern Ireland, we have our own Dementia Services Development Centre in Jordanstown, for which one of the aims is to lobby for dementia research. It is clear that relabeling senile dementia as Alzheimer's disease was indeed extremely successful in raising the awareness of Alzheimer's worldwide and increasing overall funding.

The medical model views dementia as a disease and the loss of 'normality' of those affected and focuses on the neuropathology of the brain and the declining cognitive functioning of the individual. Because of its mainly scientific base, the medical model does not take into account the concepts of the lived experience of the person with dementia and the social, environmental, family, and humane factors (Cooper 2001).

Drugs are more commonly prescribed now, and they have their place – albeit limited as far as cognitive enhancers go. The purpose of prescribing drugs is to delay for as long as possible severe memory loss or slow down the progression of symptoms or possible decline leading to dependency. The Standard Medical Advisory Committee (1998) stated that 'at present too little is known about the duration of benefit'. Further controlled trials are urgently needed to determine how long prescribing is justified, even in patients who benefit initially. The Chief Nursing Officers Review of Mental Health Services (DOH 2006) outlines that mental-health nursing needs to move away from the traditional medical model and adopt a focused biopsychosocial approach. One GP commented to the author that he got frustrated when nurses rang him for medication to sedate patients who were diagnosed with dementia and experiencing challenging behaviour. 'Would it not have been better to find the cause?' he commented. The author, in practice, has also observed situations where undetected physical health problems led to challenging behaviour in patients experiencing dementia. Nursing has been based on the structure of the nursing process and nursing models. Assessment is the first of many interventions and described as 'the ongoing process of gathering information' (Willis and Ford 2001). The key to achieving high standards of nursing interventions is through assessment of both physical and mental health within the biopsychosocial framework. This would result in reducing the risk of deterioration in health and level of dependency.

The role of the community nurse is to assess, monitor, and provide support for the individual, carer, and family, to recommend and implement as appropriate various psychological treatments such as cognitive training and memory enhancement. In order to achieve good patient outcomes, early detection and intervention is vital (Barlow, cited in Marshall 2005).

With the ever-increasing ageing population, the government decided to withdraw long-stay hospital beds, and the Community Care Act (DOH 1990) was slowly implemented. The emphasis is now on keeping patients in the community for as long as possible, but the time may come when the person can no longer be cared for safely at home.

Admission to a private nursing/care home may be the only option. Instead of large wards for people experiencing dementia, they now are admitted to more personal surroundings, mainly in the private sector, especially when they need twenty-four-hour care. Nursing care homes are now better resourced with trained staff who uphold the freedom of choice for patients with their families, are involved in decision-making, and have more personal control over their lifestyles, based on an effective risk assessment (NMC 2002). Nursing care homes have become more focused on the activities of daily living, family, and community involvement and management systems to guide the delivery of care.

Training in dementia is now promoted within nursing homes. The 'Yesterday Today and Tomorrow' training, which is a six-week course covering all aspects of dementia care, is provided to all staff, including ancillary staff (Alzheimer's Society 2002).

The author works in a private nursing care home, and as a result of current training recognised that the environment needed to be enriched to increase the perceptual senses of the residents. 'Enriching the sensory experience does not necessarily require the purchase of expensive equipment' (Willocks 1994).

Under the guidance of the dementia specialist, the author introduced a coffee percolator into the main body of the unit, so that residents can help themselves to a cup when they want, with the intention that the aroma would be stimulating.

It was also noted that at tea time, residents were more anxious, therefore by separating the large dining room into half dining and the other half a sitting area with wicker chairs and settees that were already in the home, another new dining room was prepared, and the whole dining experience became more relaxed. Tablecloths were purchased, flowers placed on top, and full settings for each meal, including salt, pepper, sauces, and serviettes, were provided.

This improvement to the dining experience made mealtimes more enjoyable for residents, visitors, and staff. The author is of the belief that these changes and also meeting the required Regulation and Quality Improvement Authority (RQIA) 2005 standards has greatly enhanced the quality of life for people experiencing dementia.

The promotion of relabeling senile dementia to Alzheimer's disease has helped to make the illness more acceptable to the general public. As a result, funding was made available for research about the illness, as it is hoped a cure could be found or at least the chance to give the patient a better quality of life.

The world of dementia care has come a long way from the bad old days of senile dementia. The environment has changed from the institution to more homely surroundings, and there is not the stigma attached to the illness that there used to be. Treatment is individualized and aims to meet care needs in a holistic way. Standards are now set to ensure good quality of care (RQIA 2003).

Drugs used in the treatment of dementia assist in prolonging cognitive ability, and thus the person has a better quality of life for a longer period of time.

There is now a greater understanding of the feelings and fears that people with Alzheimer's experience, and with the training given to all staff, it should now be hoped to help the patient cope with the illness.

With the above improvements, it may not be inevitable that dementia will decline into dependency. Kitwood (1997) pointed out 'there is a difference between a person dying with dementia and a person dying from dementia'.

Footnote: Written after assignment but worthy of thought now.

Some figures issued by Alzheimer's Society UK 2015:

- By 2015, there will be 850,000 people with dementia in the UK.
- There are 40,000 younger people with dementia.
- There are 25,000 people with dementia from black and minority ethnic groups.
- There will be one million people with dementia in the UK by 2025.
- Two-thirds of people with dementia are women.

- The proportion of people with dementia doubles for every five-year age group.
- One in six people aged eighty and over have dementia.
- Sixty thousand deaths a year are directly attributable to dementia.
- Delaying the onset of dementia by five years would reduce the deaths directly attributable to dementia by 30,000 a year.
- The financial cost of dementia to the UK is twenty-six billion pounds sterling per annum.
- There are 670,000 carers of people with dementia in the UK.
- Family carers of people with dementia save the UK eleven billion pounds sterling a year.
- Eighty per cent of people living in care homes have a form of dementia or severe memory problems.
- Two-thirds of people with dementia live in the community, while one-third live in a care home.
- Only 44 per cent of people with dementia in England, Wales, and Northern Ireland receive a diagnosis.

Person-Centred Care (PCC) University Module

Below is part of my assignment for university, based on PCC (person-centred care).

The focus of this study is to examine and explore to what extent the concept of PCC, person-centred care meets the care needs of people with dementia and those who care for them.

I am a nursing sister in a nursing home, caring for people who experience dementia, and I wish to show how PCC is provided in my place of work for both the resident and the carer in the nursing home environment.

To answer the above question, I will study books written by people who are experts in the field of dementia, articles from various peer-reviewed journals, Internet articles, television and from my own work experience.

This is a vast subject to answer, and despite the word limitation, I will endeavour to present the key principals within the PCC philosophy on some of the areas I found relative. I hope to show nevertheless that it is possible to provide PCC in nursing homes.

For instance, I will explain the forms of dementia, the challenge for planners of services, and the old and new culture of care.

I will investigate what PCC really means, including personhood, malignant psychology, validation, and attachment theory – what the needs of the person are and how to interpret them without resorting to lies as a first response.

I will also examine how staff is supported in providing PCC and finally discuss how dementia can be promoted in the future.

According to the International Classification of Diseases (ICD 10 2002), dementia is defined as

> A syndrome due to disease of the brain, usually of a chronic or progressive nature in which there is disturbance of multiple higher cortical function including memory, thinking, orientation, comprehension, calculation, language and judgement. Consciousness is not clouded. The impairment of cognitive function is commonly accompanied and occasionally preceded by deterioration in emotional control, social behaviour or motivation.

Dementia is predominantly a disorder of the very elderly (McKeith and Fairbairn 2001). This is not always the case, as it is recorded that Frau Auguste D, the first person with a written-up clinical diagnosis of dementia by Dr Alois Alzheimer, was only fifty-five years of age when she died (Maurer, Volk, et al. 1997).

There are numerous forms of dementia. The most common one is Alzheimer's disease, sometimes referred to as dementia of the Alzheimer's type (DAT). Other well-recognised forms of dementia include Dementia with Levy Bodies, Vascular, and Pick's disease, to mention just a few.

The growth of the elderly population poses great challenges to services, and provision must be made for the changing structures of society.

The demography landscape is changing mainly due to the increase in life expectancy and lowering birth rates. The UK census (2001) revealed that the life expectancy of a female born in the UK in 2001 was eighty years of age, with males expected to live seventy-five years. It predicts by the year 2014, the number of people aged sixty-five years will outnumber those aged less than sixteen years of age. This is a great challenge for planners of services, in order to meet the future needs of people with dementia. The prevalence of dementia and particularly Alzheimer's disease increases with age; thus, age is the biggest risk, and dementia is emerging as a major health and social-services dilemma (Bowie and Takrita 2004).

Research from Fox (1989) showed that 'senile dementia' was the fourth-leading cause of death in the United States.

Katzman and Karasu (as cited in Fields 1975) suggested that establishing dementia as an illness with a high mortality rate, rather than an aspect of ageing, would aid attempts at greater funding. This made dementia more acceptable to the public, as the stigma (Goffman 1963) of mental disease was reduced, and research might find a cure.

The old culture of care relied on the medical model, whereby unnecessary medication was used to control the patient, thus reduced dementia to a biomedical phenomenon (Kitwood 1996), was task-driven, and used techniques including restraints both chemical and physical (Jensen 1998).

This type of care devalued the person with dementia as a whole. The patients were admitted to institutions (insane asylums), away from public view, with little or no privacy, dignity, stimulation, or family input (Goffman 1963). These institutions had large dormitories and lacked in social, recreational, and bathing facilities.

Michael Meacher (1972) in his famous study of residential homes suggested that the social psychology and general arrangements were virtually sufficient in themselves to 'drive people demented'.

The new culture of care integrates a combination of biological and psychological philosophy with social theories, whereby PCC focuses on independence, well-being, and empowerment of individuals and families (Mitchell 1999). Younger (2000) stated that this 'enables the person to feel supported, valued and socially confident'. PCC has resulted in the concept of the 'person' being at the centre of cultured care, which has changed the focus of how people are viewed and therefore treated. Kitwood (1997) outlined that the 'person' is of the utmost importance when dealing with someone experiencing dementia.

This change in the culture of care focuses on the holistic care of the person experiencing dementia and is based on different findings on the works of Marshall (1988) and Gilleard (1984) to name a few. They showed it was more acceptable to focus on the whole person and on the real-life experiences of that person, rather than focusing alone on dementia as a disease. Chester et al. (1999) also stated that PCC centres on the abilities but not on the losses and focuses on the remaining cognitions, emotions, and capabilities of the person. He emphasised the need to value the person within the content of gender, culture, relationships, and society.

In order to provide PCC, the person must have holistic assessments, which also involve their carers (Pritchard 1999). These assessments are carried out in a nonjudgmental way, to build trust and rapport (Martin 2000). Individual care plans are developed based on assessed needs. Continual assessments and care plans are maintained with the involvement of carers/nursing assistants in this process (Dewing 1999). This would include the provision of alternative personal care methods, for example towel bathing (Martin 1999). This method of personal care can be used if the person refuses to have a regular shower or bath, and thus confrontation is prevented and personal hygiene is carried out.

In my area of practice, PCC is practiced through activities, which are planned and developed following the PCC assessment to suit the abilities of the person. If the person does not like music, for example, then an alternative activity would be supplied, such as art. This would be based on their personal history and what the person would like to do at that present time.

According to Kitwood (1997), personhood is 'a standing or status that is bestowed upon human beings, by others, in the context of relationships and social being, implying recognition, respect and trust.'

Some of the qualities that are important in providing personhood within the PCC philosophy include self-awareness (Tappen R. et al. 1999), meaningful talk (Ramamathan-Abbott 1994), expressive behaviour (Dewing et al. 1999), humour and individuality (Buckwater 1995), personality, and sexuality (McLean 1994). In nursing practice, these individual qualities are elicited from the person, carer, and family, alongside holistic assessments with past history records (Clarke 2000).

It is important to maintain and strengthen the person's sense of 'personhood' (Kitwood 1997). There is evidence that people with dementia, if given the appropriate support, can experience 'rementia', that is relearning lost skills and increased cognitive clarity, despite degenerative neurological impairment (Kitwood 1995). It is at these times the person can play an important role in planning his or her own care and making decisions about appropriate support and services.

However, since Kitwood wrote his books defining the personhood of man and the malignant psychology of the past to the person, the care thinking has changed. The term *malignant psychology* refers to instances in which the person was not treated in a dignified manner but rather through such things as infantilisation, labelling, and stigmatisation (Goffman 1963) 'The term *malignant* does not, however, imply evil intent on the part of care givers; most of the work is done through kindness and good intent. The malignancy is part of our cultural heritage' (Kitwood 1997).

I have witnessed in practice occasions when malignant psychology was used, for instance, the inappropriate term 'wanderer' being used to describe a person experiencing dementia. I have explained to the staff the meaning of the person's actions, that the person is walking around in an attempt to achieve his or her aim (Hughes, Julian, et al. 2006).

A possible way to avoid engaging in malignant positioning and malignant psychology and thus engage in PCC is to consider the meaning of a simple yet profound statement uttered by the late Christopher Reeve. Reeve had considered suicide after his accident, which left him paralysed from the neck down. When asked why he changed his mind, he said, 'I had to stop being a patient and start being a person.' This shows us no matter how severely disabled a person is, his or her life can be improved by giving the proper kind of support to enjoy positive, valued social identities far beyond the restrictions imposed by that of the illness (Hughes et al. 2006).

People experiencing dementia are continually finding themselves in situations that are 'strange' to them, and this is very frightening (Miesen 1995). Specific needs within PCC need to be met if we are to help the person experiencing dementia, and Kitwood (1997) specified five needs: bonding, comfort, inclusion, occupation, and identity.

Bonding

Early childhood provides a sense of security and is essential for the human to function. It is suggested by Kitwood (1997) that in the person with dementia, the need for attachment is just as strong as in early childhood. Bowlby (1972) argues that attachment needs remain important throughout life, and he has used attachment theory to explain that dementia is a strange and frightening disease, that great fears are experienced, and if attachment needs are not met, it can result in failure to thrive and – in extreme cases – even death.

Comfort

Spending quality time with someone who is obviously distressed.

Inclusion

Being involved in the everyday functions of the home and social life. If the need is not met, a person is likely to decline and retreat into himself.

Occupation

Taking part in meaningful activities. Providing a project, whether work or play, which draws on the person's abilities and powers. If a person is deprived of occupation, her abilities shrink, and she loses self-esteem.

Identity

This is conveyed by others onto a person. It is essential to know past history to know how to convey and provide empathy for the person.

Fiel (1993) recommended validation techniques on how to help people come to terms with their fears of the disease and have the aforementioned needs met. She advocated that a person who is trained in the different techniques of validation can talk the person through and thus help them resolve problems, which may prevent them deteriorating.

For example, a resident in the home where I work kept saying to everyone, 'Can I have a start?' Unless the staff had read his past history and understood his employment and life history, they would not know what he was asking for. This resident had worked all his life in the construction industry. In order for him to get a job, he had to go to a building site on a Monday morning at 6 a.m. and ask for 'a start', which meant he was available for employment. This resident was looking for work. I spent time talking to this resident about his life's work, and I planned structured activities for him to fulfil his occupational needs.

It is vital that staff is trained in dementia care, so they are able to understand and respond to a person when that person says, for example, 'I want to go to work' or 'see my mother'. Wood-Mitchel (2006) questions whether telling lies is an appropriate response in instances such as the aforementioned. James et al. (2006) suggest that the truth should be used as the first option to fulfil the need. A further three options, e.g., activities or the giving of a doll, should be attempted to divert the person, and if still unsuccessful, only then consider using a therapeutic lie. Jackson (2005) suggests that if a lie has fewer side effects than offering medication to solve the problem, then lying is the better alternative. It is hoped that by following this in practice within dementia care, lying will not be taken for granted but is prevented, addressed, and out in the open (Kitwood 1997).

In the environment of a nursing care home, it may be more difficult to carry out PCC, especially if, for example, staff routines, mealtimes, and toileting times are regimental. This places the staff in conflict with the very essence of 'person-centeredness' (Williams 1999). It is much easier to provide PCC in a client-oriented nursing home environment where freedom of choice for activities, meals, toileting, and bedtimes is given. It was noted that decreased verbal agitation resulted, the person slept better, and staff were less stressed and more tolerant of residents' behaviour (Mathews 1996).

In practice, PCC is evaluated by the outcomes that are achieved for the person. PCC philosophy incorporates consistent reviewing of care and interventions that keeps the person central at all times.

In providing PCC in the home that I work in, the role of the carer/nursing assistant is very important, as they are the people who are closest to the client in terms of providing personal care and communication. This is a very demanding and often stressful but rewarding work.

The need for training to promote PCC and to support staff in their work is vital. The training is provided under the umbrella of the Alzheimer's Society, which is an intense six-week course called Yesterday Today and Tomorrow (Alzheimer's Society 2002), which covers all aspects of dementia care. The nursing assistants/carers, when they finish the course, are more relaxed in dealing with the everyday problems of work, understand the principles of good communication (Killick 2001), and are aware of how the environment could enhance communication or detract from it.

Carers in nursing homes have the added role of supporting the families of the person, as the family sometimes feel that caring for a family member at home is considered a moral obligation (Baldwin and Twigg 1991). Within PCC, the carer develops good relationships with the family and gets their involvement, for example with supplying past history, likes and dislikes of the patient. Various organisations, both local and national, aim to support both carers and people with dementia, the Alzheimer's Society and Age Concern being the most recognised.

In looking to the future with ourselves in mind, we must educate the youth. It is my opinion that dementia should be part of the national curriculum in schools.

The Alzheimer's Society is the leading campaigner for dementia. I would advocate that we support our local branch, as they in turn support the people with dementia and their families. Alzheimer's Europe 'Making Dementia a Public Health Priority' is dedicated to the public-health impact of Alzheimer's disease and the other forms of dementia in Europe. It is hoped that by going 'Europe', support from key members of the European Parliament will bring action to making dementia a political priority.

In conclusion, I have attempted to answer the question to what extent does a person-centred philosophy meet the care needs of people with dementia and those who care for them.

In preparation for the article, I have read numerous books written by experts in this field, including peer-reviewed journals, the Internet, television, and my own personal experience of working in a nursing home with people who experience dementia. From research, I have defined what dementia is and whom it affects, and the evidence shows the scale of the problem for the services to be provided, that we must plan for the future.

I have shown practical evidence of PCC in the nursing home environment and explained the qualities of personhood. It is generally agreed by all the authors that the needs of the person is central to bestowing recognition, respect, and trust. This is through learning the person's past history, helping them when agitated through validation within the new culture of care without resorting to lies in the first instance, or engaging in malignant psychology, of the old culture of care in meeting residents' needs.

It is evident that carers need PCC to help them provide good-quality care, and they need support to do this. I have shown that training provided by the nursing care home gives carers and nursing assistants insight into dementia and how to respond to situations as they arise.

I have demonstrated how I, in practice, utilise PCC philosophy by using the nursing process, which outlines individual needs and includes the family, keeping the person and their needs central at all times.

In planning for the future, I have suggested that the media helped immensely in campaigning to get recognition, respect, and finance for AIDS victims; maybe the campaigners for dementia should get the media to help promote dementia, alongside charities and government bodies.

I feel I have shown that the care needs of people with dementia and those who care for them are greatly enhanced by the implementation of the concept of person-centred philosophy. It is my opinion that PCC is not a matter of choice but a necessity in ensuring positive-valued social identities far beyond the possible restrictions of dementia.

Epilogue

Thank you for reading about my experiences and observations I have gained throughout my working years. As I said at the beginning of this book, I primarily started this writing to inform my own family, just in case I should develop dementia of any type myself. I now feel if anyone who has read this book has the same concern about their future, now is a good time to document your wishes and save it in a safe place.

Remember, it is the small things that count, and it may make such a difference to our future care. For example, I wear bed socks in bed to prevent my feet getting cold during the night, as the cold causes my feet and legs to have cramps. I have tried other methods to treat this, but the socks are the simplest treatment, and it works. I also like the feeling of the socks. My family would not be aware of this problem unless I tell them or write it down for the future. I like privacy for myself now, and they do not need to know now, but in the future maybe.

It is also a good idea to let your family know who you have appointed as your legal representative and where you keep this information, as well as any legal issues you want to address while you have full mental abilities.

Remember again it is usually the small things that can make a difference.

Wishing you all well.

Ann

Author References

S. Baldwin and J. Twigg, 'Women and Community Care: Reflection on a Debate', *London Routledge*, 1991.

P. Bowie and Y. Takrita, 'Epidemiology of the Dementia' in C. Curren and J.P. Wattis, *Practical Management of Dementia: A Multiprofessional Approach*. Oxford, Radcliff Medical Press, 2004.

British Medical Association, *Taking Care of the Carers*. London, BMA, 1995.

K.C. Buckwalter, L.A. Gerdner, and G.R. Hall, 'Shining Through: The Humour and Individuality of Persons with Alzheimer's Disease', *Journal Gerontol Nurse* 1995; 21:11–16.

R. Cheston and M. Bender, *Understanding Dementia. The Man with the Worried Eyes,* London and Philadelphia, Jessica Kingsley Publishers, 1999.

A. Clarke, 'Using Biography to Enhance the Nursing Care of Older People', *Brit Nurse,* 2000, 9:429–33.

Dementia Forum Northern Ireland Newsletter, Issue no. 7, 2007.

J. Dewing and S. Blackburn, 'Dementia. Part 4, Risk Management' in *Prof Nurse,* 1999, 14:803–5 and 585–88.

N. Feil, *The Validation Therapy*, Cleveland, Ohio, Edward Feil Productions, 1993.

E. Goffman, *Stigma Notes on the Management of Spoiled Identity,* Stratton, New York, 1963.

J. Hughes, et al., *Dementia Mind, Meaning, and the Person,* Biddies Ltd. King's Linn, 2006.

I C D- 10, Classification of Mental Disorders 2nd ed, Science press Ltd London, 2002.

I.A. James, et al., 'Lying to People with Dementia within Care Settings. Developing Ethic Guidelines within Care Settings', *International Journal of Geriatric Psychiatry*, 2006, 21(8)800–21.

B. Jenson, A. Hess-Zak, and S. Johnson, 'Restraint Reduction: A New Philosophy for a New Millennium', *JONA*, 1998, 28:32–38.

J. Killick and K. Allen, *Communication and the Care of People with Dementia*. Philadelphia: Open University Press, 2001.

T. Kitwood, 'Cultures of Care: Tradition and Change, in S. Benson and T. Kitwood (eds), *The New Culture of Dementia Care*, London, Hawker, 1995, pp.7–11.

――――――――, *Dementia Reconsidered*, Buckingham, Open University Press, 1997.

――――――――, 'Building Up the Mosaic of Good Practice', *Dementia Care*, 1996: 3:12–13.

T. Kitwood and K. Bredin, 'Towards a Theory of Dementia Care: Personhood and Well Being', *Ageing and Society*, 1992, 12, 269–287.

K. Lyman, 'Living with Alzheimer's Disease: The Creation of Meaning among Persons with Dementia', *J Clin Ethics*, 1998, 9:49–57.

M. Marshall, *Perspectives on Rehabilitation and Dementia*, London, Jessica Kingsley Publishers, 2005.

L.S. Martin, P. Morden, and C. Mc Dowell, 'Using the Towel Bath to Give Tender Care in Dementia: A Case Example', *Perspectives*, 1999, 23:8–11.

E. Matthews, G. Farrell, and A. Blackmore, 'Effects of an Environmental Manipulation Emphasizing Client-Centered Cares on Agitation and Sleep in Dementia Sufferers in a Nursing Home', *Journal Adv Nurs*, 1996, 24:439–47.

K. Maurer, S. Volk, and H. Gerbaldo, 'Auguste D and Alzheimer's Disease', *Lancet*, 1997, 349 (no. 9064). 1546–1549.

A. Mc Lean, 'What Kind of Love Is This?', *Sciences,* New York, 1994, 34:36–9.

I. McKeith, and A. Fairgurn, 'Biomedical and Clinical Perspectives', in C. Cantley (ed.), *A Handbook of Dementia Care,* Buckingham, Open University Press, 2001, 7–25.

M. Meacher, *Taken for a Ride.* London, Longmans, 1972.

B. Miesen, 'Alzheimer's Disease, the Phenomenon of Parent Fixation and Bowlby's Attachment Theory', *International Journal of Geriatric Psychiatry,* 1995, 8, 147–153.

B. Miesen, (eds) *Caregiving in Dementia*, vol. 1 London, Routledge.

R. Mitchell, *Commentary, Int Journal Ger Psy,* 1999, 14:107–8.

B. Napier, 'Diversity and Aging: Cultural Understanding as a Powerful Force in Patient-Centered Healing', *Home Care Provider,* 1998, 3:38–40.

E. Prithard, 'Dementia. Part 2: Person-Centered Assessment', *Prof Nurse,* 1999, 14:655–60.

V. Ramanathan-Abbott, 'International Differences in Alzheimer's Discourse: An Examination of AD Speech across Two Audiences', *Language in Society,* 1994, 23:31–58.

R. Tappen, C. Williams, and S. Fishman, 'Persistence of Self in Advanced Alzheimer's Disease', IMAGE: *J Nursing Scholarship,* 1999, 31:121–5.

B. Williams, D. Cattell, and M. Greenwood, 'Exploring "Person-Centeredness": User Perspectives on a Model of Social Psychiatry', Health Soc Care Community, 1999, 7:475–82.

A. Wood-Mitchell, 'Lying to People with Dementia: Sparking the Debate', *Journal of Dementia Care,* Nov/Dec 2006, page 31, accessed 20 Nov 2007.

www.Crossroads.org.uk. 'Caring for Carers', accessed 25 Nov 2007.

www.AlzheimersSociety.org, 'Yesterday Today and Tomorrow', accessed 4/10/2007.

www.Alzheimer's.org.uk/uk/news and campaign/policy watch/demography. 'A Policy Position Paper – Demography', accessed 20 October 2007.

D. Younger and G. Martin, 'Dementia Care Mapping: An Approach to Qualify Audit of Services for People with Dementia in Two Health Districts', *Adv Nurs,* 2000, 32:1206–12.

About the Author

Nurse Ann is a retired nurse with over thirty years' experience in the Dementia/Alzheimer's care sector, based in Northern Ireland. She is happily married for over forty years with four grown children who live nearby.

Her nursing qualifications and experience include general nursing training, training with vulnerable adults, courses in abuse, health and safety, moving and handling, challenging behaviour, pain, COSHE, and Training for Trainers, an Alzheimer's course whereby she has been trained to train all staff in the understanding and caring for Alzheimer's patients. She has an Alzheimer's University module in Dementia care.

She believes that this training plus her on-the-floor experience qualifies her to complete this book.

Like Florence Nightingale, she feels nursing hands on is still the best means of caring for and knowing people's needs.

About the Book

This book is an information guide on how to recognise a good nursing/care home for people suffering from Dementia and in particular Alzheimer's-type Dementia.

You will learn what you need to know before you visit your first home, what questions to ask the manager, and what to look out for when visiting the home.

The book deals with areas such as location, decor of unit, trained staff, nursing care, activities, and abuse, which are all factors important when choosing the home. Also discussed is challenging behaviour and the benefits of admitting the Alzheimer's patient to the home, plus much more.

Dementia and Person-Centred Care (PCC) are discussed in detail.

The aim of this book is to inform the uninformed. It is written in a step-by-step approach, in layman's terms. to help you decide which home to choose for your loved one who suffers from Dementia. This can be done effectively by walking around the home, observing, and knowing what questions to ask.